# Healthcare Using Marine Organisms

# Healthcare Using Marine Organisms

## Se-Kwon Kim

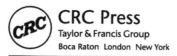

**CRC Press**
Taylor & Francis Group
Boca Raton  London  New York

CRC Press is an imprint of the
Taylor & Francis Group, an **informa** business

CRC Press
Taylor & Francis Group
6000 Broken Sound Parkway NW, Suite 300
Boca Raton, FL 33487-2742

First issued in paperback 2023

© 2018 by Taylor & Francis Group, LLC
CRC Press is an imprint of Taylor & Francis Group, an Informa business

No claim to original U.S. Government works

**Visit the Taylor & Francis Web site at**
**http://www.taylorandfrancis.com**

**and the CRC Press Web site at**
**http://www.crcpress.com**

ISBN 13: 978-1-032-65294-8 (pbk)
ISBN 13: 978-1-138-29538-4 (hbk)
ISBN 13: 978-1-315-10046-3 (ebk)

DOI: 10.1201/b22344

# Contents

# Preface

In recent years, interest in food and health has been gradually increasing, as the modern society has become an aging one. The dissemination of information on food and health is important, as people are becoming prone to disease development due to the deterioration of the environment. Although there is a growing interest in preventive medicine versus treatment-centered medicine in the medical field, few drugs to date can be called preventive drugs. To prevent diseases such as cancer, arteriosclerosis, and diabetes, functional foods should be actively introduced as preventive medicine.

Foods may exhibit completely different functions in a living body, depending on whether their components are simple substances providing energy and nutrition or valid *functional entities*. For example, although the natural biopolymer, chitin, is contained in the shells of crabs and shrimps in large quantities, it cannot be absorbed even if it is ingested because chitin does not degrade in the gastrointestinal tract of the human body. However, when chitin is transformed into chitosan (the deacetylated form of chitin) and degraded by enzymes, it becomes oligosaccharides, which are easily absorbed in the living body where they carry out diverse physiological functions.

In other words, the term *bioactive substances* refer to the molecules that promote the functions of the human body and correct abnormal pathological conditions. These substances are essential for the human body to lead a healthier life. The search for bioactive substances from natural resources has been focused majorly on terrestrial biological resources, because humans have long been growing terrestrial biological resources that have been in use as medicines for ages, and terrestrial biological resources can easily be mass-produced as raw material resources. Land resources have been so extensively studied to the extent that only a few species of living organisms are yet to be examined.

Accordingly, the developed countries are now focusing and investing actively in marine living resources, which have been left unexplored thus far. The studies in this field are progressively increasing in number due to advancements in related fields, along with the development of collection, aquaculture, and analysis technologies. As at least 80% of species of all living organisms live in the ocean, the ocean remains a repository of inexhaustible resources based on its diversity of species of living organisms.

The Chinese medical book, 中華本草 (*Chinese Medical Herbs*), contains records of the use of at least 200 species of marine life in Chinese medicine or folk remedies of ancient times, indicating that the use of marine bioactive substances (natural substances) has been done since ancient times. Oceans have environments that form unique ecosystems, different from those on the land. To survive in the competition of survival of the fittest, the secondary metabolites of marine organisms (especially those lacking adequate physical defense abilities) have chemical characteristics different from those of terrestrial organisms and demonstrate unique chemical defenses. When these substances are administered to humans or other mammalian animals, they often lead to strong physiological activity. Therefore, studies intending to elucidate new medicines of marine origin for preventing diseases have been in the limelight recently.

Our marine biochemistry laboratory has been conducting research for more than 40 years on the development of high value-added, new bioactive materials of marine origin. We have already published interesting outcomes on the activities of such materials, such as anticancer, anti-aging, antihypertension, antidiabetes, sleep-promoting, anti-allergy, and improved hair growth, in reputed international journals. I take this opportunity to introduce the outcomes by writing this book, which will help the public to alleviate various diseases. Advertisements regarding healthy foods in print and electronic media are generally presented without a proper scientific background. We presume that consuming these health foods without any proper justification poses many problems. Unfortunately, consumers are easily lured in many cases because they lack expert knowledge of relevant topics. In this book, a basic knowledge of various regular lifestyle diseases and a concrete explanation using experimental data are introduced. Technical terms have been explained to help readers understand the terms appearing in this book.

**Prof. Se-Kwon Kim**

# Acknowledgments

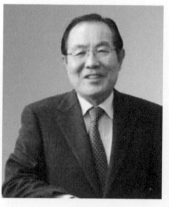 **Dr. Dong-Han Yoon,** the CEO of Kolmar Korea Co, Ltd., established Kolmar Korea in 1990 and introduced a new business model, the original design manufacturer network, to supply cosmetics, pharmaceuticals, and health functional foods.

In recent years, Dr. Yoon recognized the value of under-utilized marine resources, and felt the need to develop products through researches that can utilize them more effectively. He invited me as a research adviser and dedicated himself to publishing technical books emphasizing the scientific value of marine life and related research.

With his help, this book has been published, providing many readers with the knowledge of how scientific values of marine life can enhance human health.

I would like to thank him for continuous support and encouragement to publish this book with CRC Press.

Further, I thank CRC Press for their continuous encouragement and suggestions. I also thank Prof. Jayachandran Venkatesan, who worked with me throughout the course of this book project.

**Prof. Se-Kwon Kim**
*Korea Maritime and Ocean University*
*Busan, South Korea*

# Author

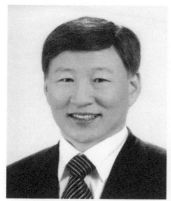

**Se-Kwon Kim,** PhD, is presently working as a distinguished professor in Korea Maritime and Ocean University, Busan, South Korea and research advisor of Kolmar Korea Co, Ltd., South Korea. He has worked as a distinguished professor at the Department of Marine Bio Convergence Science and Technology and director of Marine Bioprocess Research Center (MBPRC) at Pukyong National University, Busan, South Korea.

He earned his MSc and PhD degrees from Pukyong National University and conducted his postdoctoral studies at the Laboratory of Biochemical Engineering, University of Illinois at Urbana–Champaign, Champaign, Illinois. Later, he became a visiting scientist at the Memorial University of Newfoundland, St. John's, Canada and University of British Colombia, Vancouver, Canada.

Dr. Kim served as president of the Korean Society of Chitin and Chitosan in 1986–1990 and the Korean Society of Marine Biotechnology in 2006–2007. To the credit for his research, he won the best paper award from the American Oil Chemists' Society in 2002. Dr. Kim was also the chairman for *7th Asia-pacific Chitin and Chitosan Symposium*, which was held in South Korea in 2006. He was the chief editor of the *Korean Society of Fisheries and Aquatic Science* during 2008–2009. In addition, he is the board member of the International Society of Marine Biotechnology Associations (IMBA) and the International Society of Nutraceuticals and Functional Food (ISNFF).

His major research interests are investigation and development of bioactive substances from marine resources. His immense experience of marine bioprocessing and mass-production technologies for marine bioindustry is the key asset of holding majorly funded marine bioprojects in Korea. Furthermore, he expended his research fields up to the development of bioactive materials from marine organisms for their applications in oriental medicine, cosmeceuticals, and nutraceuticals. To this date, he has authored around 650 research papers, 70 books, and 120 patents.

*chapter one*

# Functional food and disease prevention

Currently, most people are living in semi-unhealthy conditions such that they can neither be termed as particularly ill nor completely healthy. The incidences of chronic degenerative diseases, such as stroke, arteriosclerosis, hypertension, cancer, diabetes, chronic hepatic diseases, chronic gastroenterocolitis, and chronic cardiac disease, are increasing drastically and in many instances are proving fatal. Furthermore, these health issues are turning into social problems owing to a higher incidence not only among adults but also in children. Medicines are largely used with an aim to treat diseases caused by infectious agents during undernourished conditions, which act as one of the susceptibility factors. However, the individuals who have acquired a chronic degenerative disease can hardly recover from deteriorating health conditions. Therefore, preventive medicine is indispensable to maintain and improve individuals' current health so as to prevent them from contracting such diseases. It is well known that many changes in the health conditions of people these days are consequences of alterations in lifestyle and living environment, especially with respect to diet.

The *National Population and Housing Census* report commissioned by the South Korean government in 2012 was statistically analyzed to find out the areas among 17 counties with a 1.0% or a higher amount of people aged at least 80 years. According to the statistics, Jeju-do demonstrated the highest longevity rate (1.03%), and was followed by Jeonnam (0.79%), Jeonbuk (0.66%), Gyeongbuk (0.65%), and Gyeongnam (0.61%) in that order, whereas Incheon (0.22%) showed the lowest longevity rate. The longevity rates of Seoul and Busan were 0.23% and 0.28%, respectively. In general, large cities displayed lower longevity rates than did the villages involved in agriculture and fishing. Although the reason for this finding is not clear, environmental factors and dietary culture are assumed to be the most important causes. Notably, the effects of these are exemplified by Japanese people, who have the world's highest longevity rate. Unlike other island countries, Japan has coastal areas with abundant plankton and is the primary producer in the oceanic food chain. Plankton grow more easily due to the meeting of cold and warm currents, which occurs near Japan. In other words, Japan is a country equipped with favorable conditions and an abundance of marine resources, the consumption of which bestows various benefits on the Japanese people. This is supported by the fact that Japan is the country with the highest longevity rate in the world.

The Japan Prevention and Cancer Research Institute epidemiologically investigated the causes of 265,000 deaths of Japanese individuals for 17 years, and the results indicated that the higher the frequency of fish meal consumed, the longer the people lived. It has also been shown that an increase in the morbidity and mortality rates of various adult diseases can be suppressed with the intake of fish and shellfish (Table 1.1).

In 400 B.C., Hippocrates, the father of medicine, argued that diseases could be cured by food, and that the right choice of food would lead to health benefits. In addition, modern medicine reveals that chronic degenerative diseases are closely related with the kind of food we consume every day and, therefore, chronic degenerative diseases are termed as *foodborne diseases*. It has been demonstrated that at least 40 kinds of nutrients are necessary for good physical health, including 16 kinds of vitamins and 17 kinds of minerals, in addition to essential amino acids. Since the roles of these nutrients in the body are diverse and physiologically related with each other, even the deficiency of one of them leads to a collapse of the nutritional balance, thereby ruining the individual's health. A proper understanding of the knowledge of food and nutrition is essential, which is actively reflected by the human dietary lifestyle. Therefore, it is easier for many people to prevent foodborne diseases by maintaining a

*Table 1.1* Mortality rates according to fish and shellfish intake frequencies (relative risk)

| Cause of death | Consumption of fishery products | | | | Relative risk[a] |
| --- | --- | --- | --- | --- | --- |
| | Every day | Frequently | From time to time | Never | |
| Total deaths | 1 | 1.07 | 1.12 | 1.32 | 9.134 |
| Cerebrovascular disease | 1 | 1.08 | 1.1 | 1.1 | 4.541 |
| Heart disease | 1 | 1.09 | 1.13 | 1.24 | 3.919 |
| Hypertension | 1 | 1.55 | 1.89 | 1.79 | 4.143 |
| Myoclonus | 1 | 1.21 | 1.3 | 1.74 | 3.768 |
| Stomach cancer | 1 | 1.04 | 1.04 | 1.44 | 2.144 |
| Liver cancer | 1 | 1.03 | 1.16 | 2.62 | 2.109 |
| Uterine cancer | 1 | 1.28 | 1.71 | 2.37 | 4.142 |
| Survey subjects (person) | 1,412,740 | 2,186,368 | 203,945 | 28,943 | |

[a] The higher number indicates the relative higher risk of death.

healthy lifestyle. To this end, not only South Korea, but also other coun-tries around the world are doing their best to identify physiologically important functional components that have not yet been found in food.

## 1.1   The concept of food is changing

The modern society is represented by an era of glutenization, individual-ization, and diversification. These days, both the quantitative and qualita-tive aspects of food are changing. Advancements in the modern medical system have resulted in remarkable improvements in the human physique and average human life span. With respect to the nutritional aspect, the incidence of diseases such as cancers, circulatory system conditions such as arteriosclerosis, and heart problems, are increasing due to an excessive intake of high-calorie fats (such as animal fat). The earlier thought that diseases should be medically treated has changed and has led many to think that prevention should take precedence over treatment. It has been recognized that a change in the pattern and improvement of the dietary lifestyle are important for the prevention of diseases. Based on nutritional science, food chemistry, and physiology, people have gradually recog-nized the fact that the intake of food components suitable for human nutrition is extremely important. Gradually, the emphasis has shifted to the functionality of food and the fact that in addition to the nutrition and palatability of food, the importance of basic physiological activity of the human body is essential.

At times when food was scarce, only nutrition was considered, and the desire to eat was strongly based on hunger. Consequently, humans started devoting their efforts to the mass production of food products. Gradually, the availability of abundant food products led humans to pur-sue palatability by choice so as to fit individuals' desires. The nutritional value of food is considered its primary function only in times of starvation, whereas the selective and secondary functions of food began to appear in environments once the food became more abundant. The biomodulating functions of food can be regarded as tertiary functions (Figure 1.1).

The primary function of food refers to the nutritional value of food in human bodies, or the basic functions that are enabled by the intake of food for the maintenance of life. The secondary functions refer to the functions of specific food components that satisfy the senses of human beings. The increase in demand due to the abundance of food led to glu-tenization, which in turn resulted in an unbalanced dietary lifestyle and various related diseases. An excess of imbalance in the diet results in abnormalities in biomodulation systems. For example, the nervous system, circulatory system, endocrine system, cell differentiation system, immune system, and biodefense system can be affected by the production of toxins that can induce mutation or cause cancer. On the contrary, a balanced diet

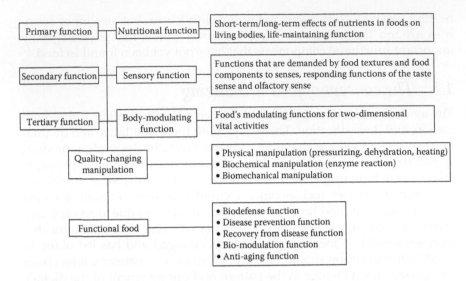

*Figure 1.1* Functions of foods.

promotes positive aspects of food components, such as antimutagenicity, anticancer properties, antioxidative activity, immune-activating properties, and cell proliferation-promoting properties. These activities serve as tertiary functions of food that can be classified as physiological functions with bio-modulating properties. The tertiary functional components can be divided into bioactive factors that express activity when the functionally active substances that present in food get directly absorbed and digested, consequently expressing the activity of these bioactive factors (Figure 1.2).

## 1.2   *Tertiary functions and health*

With the revelation of correlation between food and diseases, functional foods, which aim to prevent specific diseases, are emerging as practical social demands. When the health condition of the human body is measured with respect to the degrees of health on the vertical axis, a curve as shown in Figure 1.3 is obtained.

The points on the curve closer to the right end indicate better health conditions and the 100% health condition indicates completely healthy conditions, whereas a health condition of 0% indicates death. However, there are conditions called semi-healthy conditions that fall between 0% and 100%. Specifically, healthy and semi-healthy conditions are integral health conditions, the maintenance of which is dependent on nutrition. Even 100% healthy people should regularly consume nutrition-rich food. On the contrary, since the causes of diseases are diverse, medicines

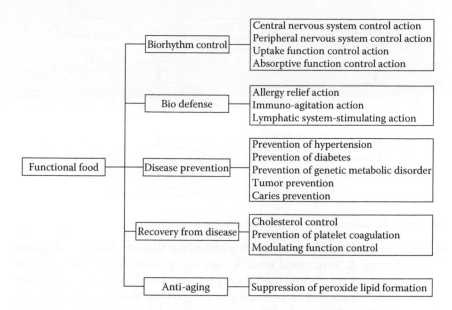

*Figure 1.2* Functions expressed by functional foods in the human body.

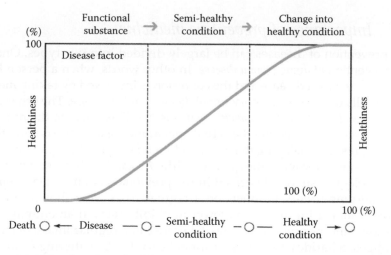

*Figure 1.3* Thoughts about health.

necessary for their treatment vary. Functional foods are necessary to convert semi-healthy conditions to the original health conditions. A semi-healthy condition is a state wherein a person has no apparent disease even when examined by a physician. Since it is too early to take medicine in such a case, the semi-healthy condition may be converted to a healthy condition with the intake of functional substances on a daily basis. For

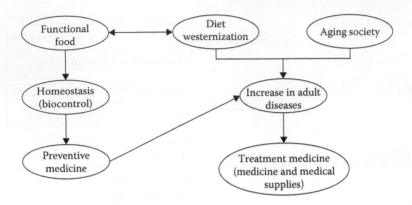

*Figure 1.4* Functional foods and adult disease prevention.

instance, in the case of a semi-healthy condition that can lead to a disposition to disease A, functional food A may be consumed. Similarly, in the case of disease B, functional food B may be consumed. As such, functional foods can be consumed to prevent diseases rather than needing to cure diseases with medicines. In this way, functional foods are equivalent to disease-specific medicines.

## 1.3   Importance of preventive medicine

The prevention of diseases can be largely divided into two types. One is the prevention *of dying from a disease*. In other words, when a person has been afflicted by a disease and the condition is improved by taking medicine, it falls under the category of *not dying from the disease*. The other one is the *prevention of the development of any disease*. This refers to the prevention of disease onset before the actual appearance of any disease. In other words, it refers to delaying the onset and increasing the life span, thereby consequently improving the quality of life. As can be observed from the epidemiological survey described in the previous section, human beings who consume fishery products on a regular basis were shown to have relatively longer life spans and lower morbidity rates. If an animal does not show cancer onset until its death because of a regular intake of chitosan oligosaccharides, the animal cannot be said to be suffering from any cancer because of the preventive measures that were taken. This method should be considered in daily lifestyle to prevent diseases such as arteriosclerosis, diabetes, senile dementia, and cancer (Figure 1.4).

Medicines or medical supplies for disease prevention are not acknowledged in any country. It is obvious that the treatment of diseases involves huge physical, temporal, and economic burdens. Therefore, preventive medicine is regarded to be of increasing importance in today's lifestyle.

*chapter two*

# What are chitin, chitosan, water-soluble chitosan, and chitosan oligosaccharides?

Chitin is a dietary fiber-based polysaccharide that is widely distributed in the natural world, including in crab and shrimp shells; the epidermis or shells of insects, such as beetles and grasshoppers; shellfishes, such as hard clams or oysters; squid bones; and the cell walls of fungi, such as mushrooms and yeast. It is a naturally occurring high-molecular-weight substance that provides protection to living organisms. Therefore, it serves a role analogous to cellulose in the vegetable kingdom. The main body of chitin is chemically a polysaccharide with a molecular weight exceeding 1,000,000 kDa in which N-acetyl-D-glucosamine residues are β-1,4-linked. Chitosan is a cationic polysaccharide and is commonly derived from chitin. It is a polysaccharide in which 2-amino-2-deoxy-D-glucose units are β-1,4-linked. Its molecular weight is less than that of chitin because it is manufactured via the deacetylation of chitin. In other words, to make chitosan, it is necessary to remove the N-acetyl group from the chitin by a process known as *deacetylation*.

Globally, the waste generated by the bodies of crustaceans such as crabs and shrimps amounts to at least 144 million tons. The quantity of chitin scrapped in seafood manufacturing processes is increasing by 120,000 tons every year. At present, approximately 3,000 tons of waste is produced in the form of chitin and chitosan. Moreover, most of the chitin, which is abundantly present, is scrapped every year as only a part of it is used. However, in recent years, studies on chitin and chitosan have been actively conducted in various countries around the world, such as Japan, South Korea, China, the United States, and various European countries. A table of contents of chitin in major food raw materials is provided in Table 2.1.

The industrial production of chitin and chitosan began in Japan in 1970 and the current output is 1,100 tons per year. In South Korea, the output is estimated to be approximately 200 tons per year. In addition, chitin and chitosan are produced in China, the United States, Poland, Norway, Taiwan, Thailand, India, and Russia. Chitin is not extensively used and is mostly employed as a precursor for manufacturing chitosan.

**Table 2.1** The chitin contents in major food raw materials (wt. %)

| Crustaceans | | Organs of fungi | |
| --- | --- | --- | --- |
| *Cancer japonicus* | 72[a3] | Hard clam shell | 6[a2] |
| Red crab | 14[a1] | Krill shell | 42[a4] |
| Yeongdeok crab | 26[a4] | Oyster shell | 4[a2] |
| Hairy crab | 18[a4] | Squid cartilage | 41[a2] |
| Sand crab | 11[a1] | | |
| *Deiratonotus cristatus* | 10[a1], 35[a2] | | |
| Alaska shrimp | 28[a4] | **Fungi** | |
| Opossum shrimp | 32[a4] | *Aspergillus niger* | 42[a5] |
| Lobster | 70[a3] | *Lactarius vellereus* | 19[a4] |
| Prawn | 25[a4] | *Mucor rouxii* | 45[a5] |
| | | *Penicillium notatum* | 19[a5] |
| | | *Saccharomyces cervisiae* | 3[a5] |
| | | *Penicillium chrysogenum* | 20[a5] |

[a1] Wet weight %
[a2] Dry weight %
[a3] Epidermis dry weight %
[a4] Total dry weight %
[a5] Dry cell wall weight %

## 2.1   What is water-soluble chitosan?

Recently, the term *water-soluble macromolecule chitosan* has been frequently seen in advertisements on television and in newspapers. We often receive queries from general consumers related to water-soluble chitosan. However, despite our explanation about water-soluble chitosan in detail, consumers are not able to comprehend its importance, probably due to a lack of relevant scientific knowledge. To understand water-soluble chitosan, the chemical structure and properties of chitosan should be known (Figure 2.1). When the acetyl group is removed from acetyl glucosamine, which is a component of chitin, it gets converted to a sugar called glucosamine. Chitosan consists of many glucosamine units linked together. However, chitosan cannot be 100% deacetylated using general methods. Therefore, chitin and chitosan exist in mixed states and are indicated as chitin/chitosan on products, where the chitosan percentage is mentioned. They are generally indicated as the degree of deacetylation,[*] specifically 50%, 70%, 80%, or 90%. This degree of deacetylation is very important for the application of chitosan.

---

[*] *Deacetylation* is simply the reverse reaction, in which an acetyl group is removed from a molecule, of *acetylation*.

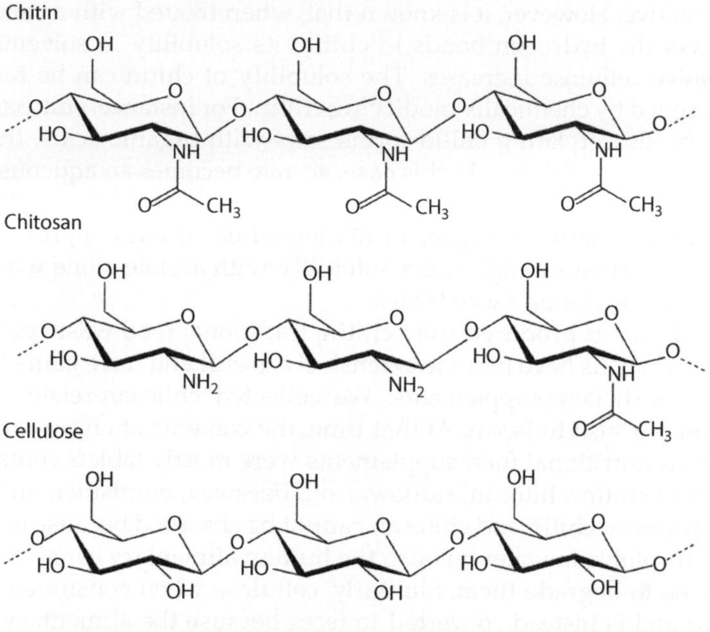

Chitin

Chitosan

Cellulose

**Figure 2.1** Structure of chitin, chitosan, and cellulose.

Quantities of chitosan at different degrees of deacetylation can be distinguished from one another to some extent by color, smell, and taste (in the case of powdered form), but chitosan cannot be delineated when it is packed into capsules. The contents of each product should be specified by mentioning the degree of deacetylation. However, in many instances, this information is not mentioned on the products. Although chitin has a very similar chemical and crystal structure to that of cellulose, its reactivity and fusibility are much different from that of cellulose. This is because it has an acetylamide group at the second carbon position of N-acetylglucosamine, a second-class hydroxyl group at the carbon-3 position, and a first class hydroxyl group (–OH) at the carbon-6 position, as shown in Figure 2.1; notably, the reactivity levels of these three different functional groups* are different from each other.

Since a hydrogen bond is formed between the hydroxyl group at the carbon-3 position and the acetamide group (CH₃CONH–) at the carbon-2 position, and the hydroxyl group at the carbon-6 position forms a hydrogen bond with a water molecule, the entire chitin molecule forms a very strong crystal structure, which is not soluble in water and therefore is

---

* *Functional group*: An atomic group with reactivity, which shows the characteristics of molecules—for instance, a hydroxyl group (–OH).

highly inactive. However, it is known that, when treated with a condition that breaks the hydrogen bonds in chitin, its solubility in solvents that can dissolve cellulose increases. The solubility of chitin can be remarkably improved by chemically modifying chitin. For instance, chitosan that is made by deacetylating chitin forms salts with organic acids, thereby exhibiting water solubility. In this case, acetate becomes an aqueous solution by a reagent that breaks hydrogen bonds, such as a dichloroacetic acid ($Cl_2CHCOOH$), until the degree of deacetylation reaches approximately 40% to 60%; it shows a high water solubility with acetate alone when the degree of deacetylation exceeds 60%.

As chitosan is produced from chitin, traditional food waste products such as crab shells have become extensively useful and have gained wide attention as dietary supplements. We collected chitosan-related products upon our visit to Japan. At that time, the contents of chitin/chitosan products as nutritional food supplements were mostly tablets containing mixtures of chitin/chitosan, safflower oil, beeswax, emulsifier, and vitamin E. However, chitin and chitosan cannot be absorbed because not only are they insoluble in water but also the human alimentary canal contains no enzyme to degrade them. Similarly, cellulose when consumed is not absorbed and is instead converted to feces because the alimentary canal lacks the enzyme to degrade it.

In humans, when proteins are ingested, they are degraded by digestive enzymes into amino acids or low-molecular-weight oligopeptides,* which are easily absorbed. Likewise, when ingested by humans, chitosan can be absorbed only after being degraded into glucosamine or low-molecular-weight oligosaccharides. Unfortunately, humans lack an enzyme that can decompose chitosan in their alimentary canal. However, many animals are different from humans. Ruminants such as cows can absorb cellulose to utilize it as an energy source because cellulose is fermented into propionic acid by microorganisms present in their stomachs. In the case of rabbits, there is a report wherein chitin and chitosan was supplied in the feed at a concentration of 2% to 5%, and 40% to 44% of chitin and chitosan was absorbed. In humans, although some amount of chitin and chitosan may be degraded and absorbed because of the enzymes that may exist in foods, such cases are rare to observe.

Chitin and chitosan are the most actively studied compounds in Japan. The emphasis is on the decomposition of chitosan using enzymes to produce oligosaccharides, which are easily absorbed by the human body. Alternatively, chitosan can be decomposed using hydrochloric acid; however, the Food Hygiene Act of Japan mentions that chitosan degraded using hydrochloric acid should not be used as a dietary supplement. This is also the case in South Korea. Even when chitosan

---

* *Oligopeptide*: A relatively small peptide consisting of about 10 amino acids.

is dissolved using organic acids* and made into a 1% solution (w/v), enzyme reactions can be hardly induced because of the high viscosity of the solution. In addition, the price of an enzyme that can degrade chitosan exceeded $300 per gram around two decades ago. In Japan, decomposing chitosan using enzymes for the mass production of oligo-saccharides was considered to be impossible. However, we developed a *continuous ultrafiltration membrane bioreactor system* in a specific research task of the Ministry of Maritime Affairs and Fisheries and succeeded in separating only the degradation product (oligosaccharides) on the basis of molecular weight by continuously circulating a certain amount of enzyme in the reactor.

When this research was presented at the Symposium of the Japanese Society for Chitin and Chitosan, the president of Fuji Bio Co., Ltd. (a company which developed and sold chitosan for the first time in Japan) visited our laboratory and proposed to invite the author to his company. The author refused the proposal by mentioning that he/she is legally bound to transfer the technology to a company only if it invests into the research fund. Recently, the term *water-soluble chitosan* has been used in Japan. It refers to chitosan that can be dissolved in water by shortening the reaction time, which is done by decomposing chitosan with enzymes or hydro-chloric acid. In fact, most chitosan oligosaccharides produced in South Korea are said to be *water-soluble chitosan*. When chitosan has been suf-ficiently degraded using enzymes to the extent that the number of polym-erized glucosamines does not exceed 100—in other words, when less than 100 glucosamine molecules have been bound together—then the chitosan is called chitosan oligosaccharides and the products of further degrada-tion can be called *water-soluble chitosan*.

Since the macromolecule form of chitosan is barely absorbed in the human body, it can absorb not only radioactive substances but also bile acid and cholesterol. Therefore, this composition of chitosan can be extremely important in dietary supplements. In addition, since macromolecule chi-tosan also binds to ingested chlorine ions and is excreted together, it can be helpful for controlling blood pressure. However, physiological actions such as immunopotentiation and anticancer activity can be shown only by absorbed chitosan oligosaccharides. Some researchers claim that chito-san is absorbed because it is not detected in the feces. However, this may be because chitosan is degraded by bacteria present in the large intestine, from where the absorption of degraded substances is very rare. Therefore, when taking chitosan-related products, having a basic knowledge about chitosan, water-soluble chitosan, chitosan oligosaccharides, and glucos-amine product contents is extremely important.

---

* *Organic acid*: An acid that contains an acidic carboxylic acid among organic compounds.

## 2.2   *What are chitosan oligosaccharides?*

Several monosaccharides such as glucose and fructose are bound together
to form products generally known as oligosaccharides. As the mechanism
of action of glycosyltransferases and hydrolases has been elucidated and
highly pure oligosaccharides have been mass-produced, oligosaccharides
with various useful functional and physiological properties have become
a topic of research these days. In addition, as new functional properties
of these oligosaccharides are revealed, diverse application fields that had
not been previously conceived in the past continue to be introduced.
Oligosaccharides are dehydrated condensates of several monosaccharides
by glycosidic bonds* and generally refer to water-soluble crystalline substances with sweet tastes. Although the length of the sugar chain of oligosaccharides has not been clearly defined, oligosaccharides generally refer
to small numbers of saccharides, which include up to 10 monosaccharides
bound together. Originally, the term, *oligo* was derived from the Greek
word *oligo*, which means minority. In recent years, however, saccharides
that include up to 100 monosaccharides bound together are considered to
be oligosaccharides in some cases.

---

* *Glycosidic bond*: A bond of two monosaccharides after the removal of one molecule of
water between the aldehyde group and the alcohol group.

# chapter three

# How to make chitin, chitosan, and chitosan oligosaccharides?

## 3.1  Manufacturing of chitin and chitosan

Chitin and chitosan are extracted from crab and shrimp shells, but these shells are composed of proteins, fats (pigment), carbohydrates (chitin), and inorganic substances such as calcium carbonate. To produce chitin from crab shells, calcium carbonate ($CaCO_3$), which is an inorganic component, must be removed first. $CaCO_3$ can be removed using hydrochloric acid and the principle for this process is as follows: Calcium carbonate, which is also called limestone, generates calcium chloride ($CaCl_2$) and carbonic acid ($H_2CO_3$) when treated with acids such as hydrochloric acid. The calcium chloride is then dissolved in water and the carbonic acid is degraded into water and carbon dioxide ($CO_2$). After removing calcium carbonate, the residue is immersed in a dilute solution of sodium hydroxide (NaOH). Proteins and pigments are degraded and chitin is obtained after the products of degradation are removed.

Chitin exists as the most abundant material in terms of quantity next to cellulose among substances present in the natural world; however, the utilization of chitin is limited due to its poor solubility and low reactivity. Chitosan can be produced from chitosan and, if solubilized in organic acids, which are weak acids, its reactivity is enhanced. This prompts the discovery of various functionalities, leading to a wide variety of utilities. To produce chitosan, the acetyl group ($CH_3CO$-) in the chitin structure is removed by heating with a solution of 40% sodium hydroxide. This is called *deacetylation*. However, producing 100% pure chitosan is a difficult task because all chemical reactions involve side reactions, and chitin and chitosan cannot be separated completely with general technology. Therefore, since chitin and chitosan exist in a mixed state, chitosan is often indicated as chitin/chitosan in many cases. However, in general, chitosan refers to the product from chitin after removal of at least 70% of acetyl groups (Figure 3.1).

High purity chitosan can be produced by increasing the concentration of the sodium hydroxide and increasing the temperature of the solution to 100°C. Lower viscosity of the chitosan solution indicates the breaking down of glycosidic bonds, leading to the production of low-molecular-weight

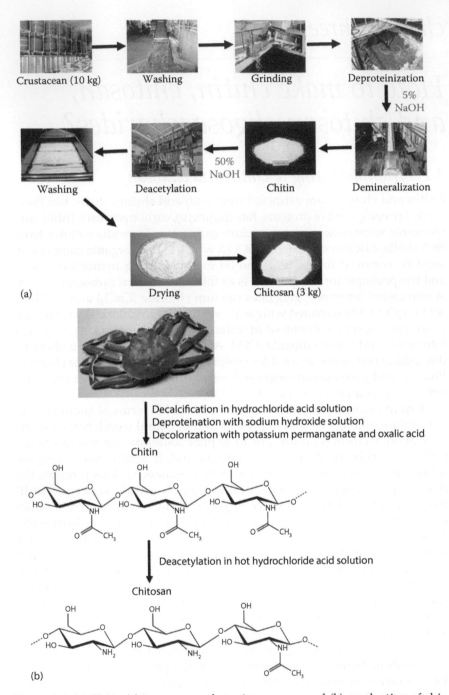

(a)

(b)

*Figure 3.1* (a) Chitin/chitosan manufacturing process and (b) production of chitin and chitosan.

chitosan. Therefore, chitosan manufacturing processes may vary depending on the purpose of use. When manufacturing chitin and chitosan, it should be noted that since the raw materials (shrimp or crab shells) are prone to quick decay, these should be processed immediately after obtaining them. Since the shells decay even when they have been left piled up only for one day, they should be dried if they are not processed immediately. If rotten shells are used as a raw material, the quality of chitin/chitosan products will be poor.

## 3.2   Oligosaccharides and their anticancer activity

As compared with chitosan, the degradation products of chitosan with the appropriate molecular weight exhibit good physiological activity. Chitosan itself does not elicit any physiological function in the human body because it is hardly absorbed even after being ingested. The structure of chitosan is similar to that of cellulose, and no enzyme degrades chitosan in the alimentary canal of the human body. Therefore, to make chitosan absorbable in the living body, it should be degraded into oligosaccharides before ingestion.

Oligosaccharides (molecular weight: 18 kDa or less) and water-soluble chitosan (molecular weight: 18 kDa or more) were orally administered to rats to identify their absorption rates in the body. The results suggested that water-soluble chitosan with a molecular weight of 22 kDa was not absorbed in the duodenum or the small intestine and that the absorption rate of oligosaccharides in the body was higher when the molecular weight was lower (Figure 3.2).

Chitooligosaccharides can be produced by two different methods: one is via the decomposition of chitin/chitosan by strong hydrochloric acid (chemical method) and the other is by using enzymes (enzymatic method). In South Korea, oligosaccharides sold in the past were produced by hydrochloric acid in most cases. When chitin is degraded using hydrochloric acid, it produces chitosan and some side reaction substances, which are harmful to the human body. It is a difficult task to completely remove the hydrochloric acid, which is used in the reaction mixture and affects the metabolism of the oligosaccharide in the body, leading to hindrance in the actions of insulin, thereby possibly causing diabetes. Therefore, the Korean Food Standards Codex of the Ministry of Health-Welfare stipulates that only those oligosaccharides that are the enzyme degradation products of chitin/chitosan may be used as food additives or health food materials.

However, since the prices of enzymes that can degrade chitin/chitosan are very high and their activity is low, the industrial production of chitin/chitosan oligosaccharides using enzyme has large economic problems. Therefore, in Japan, the products made of only chitosan per se

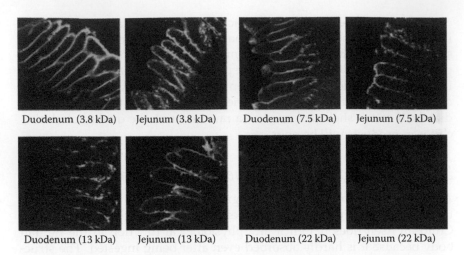

| Duodenum (3.8 kDa) | Jejunum (3.8 kDa) | Duodenum (7.5 kDa) | Jejunum (7.5 kDa) |

| Duodenum (13 kDa) | Jejunum (13 kDa) | Duodenum (22 kDa) | Jejunum (22 kDa) |

*Figure 3.2* The absorption rates of chitosan oligosaccharides and water-soluble chitosan in the bodies of rats (original magnification X100).

are distributed. There are a few products to which oligosaccharides are added; however, these oligosaccharides are not chitosan oligosaccharides but rather are obtained by decomposing starch.

Therefore, we developed a technology to produce chitosan oligosaccharides continuously using chitosanase for the first time (Figure 3.3). In order to reduce the high production cost of the enzyme consumed in large quantities during the industrial production of chitosan oligosaccharides, we attempted the development of a production system for reuse of the enzyme. To this end, we utilized an ultrafiltration membrane enzymatic reactor made by combining ultrafiltration membranes* that have been highly favored in food processes recently and a bioreactor for the production of chitosan oligosaccharides. As shown in Figure 3.3, if the reactor is filled with a chitosan solution, chitosanase is put into the reactor, and the solution is circulated with a pump, the chitosan gets degraded by the enzyme and is discharged through the ultrafiltration membrane. In this case, large particles of the chitosan degradation product and the enzyme cannot pass the ultrafiltration membrane because of their high molecular weight and continuous circulation, allowing for the decomposition reactions to progress further. The chitosan solution that can be supplied is as much as the quantity of the chitosan that was degraded in the enzymatic reactor and discharged through the ultrafiltration membrane. With this setup, chitosan oligosaccharides can be mass-produced continuously.

---

* *Ultrafiltration membrane*: A membrane that separates extremely fine particles by filtration through a filtration membrane with very small holes.

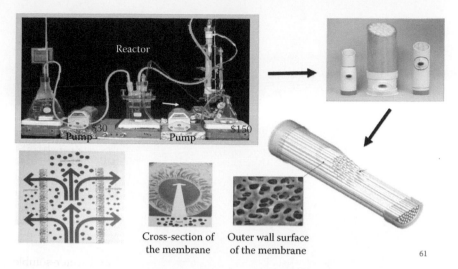

Cross-section of    Outer wall surface
the membrane       of the membrane

*Figure 3.3* A continuous chitosan oligosaccharide production process.

An advantage of the chitosan oligosaccharide production system is that chitosan oligosaccharides with desired molecular weights can be produced by using corresponding types of membranes. Since chitosan oligosaccharides show different physiological functions in the human body depending on their molecular weights, products that fit different purposes can be produced. The technology for this production system has already been transferred to an enterprise that has been producing oligosaccharide products with different molecular weights. This technology has also been provided with the Korea Good Technology (KT) certificate.

*chapter four*

# Physiological properties of chitin, chitosan, and chitosan oligosaccharides

## 4.1 Chitin/chitosan

Chitin, a natural polysaccharide, is the most widely used biomaterial as compared with other biological macromolecules. It can be extracted from crustacean shells, which are common by-products of seafood processing plants; the yearly yield of chitin is known to be approximately $1.5 \times 10^8$ tons. Although abundant quantities of by-products are generated from seafood processing plants, they have not yet been fully explored. The use of chitin is limited, possibly due to its poor solubility. However, due to its bioaffinity properties, chitin has been used in medical materials such as artificial skin and surgical suture.

However, chitosan, produced by chitin deacetylation, has a diverse range of applications. Initially, chitosan had been widely used owing to its high adsorptive properties. It can be used as a wastewater treatment agent, heavy metal absorbent, immobilized enzyme carrier, and a chromatography resin. In recent years, studies have revealed that chitosan has various physiological properties such as antimicrobial, anticancer, and immune-enhancing activities. Furthermore, it can be used in food and medicinal materials. Chitosan has agricultural applications as well: it can be added to animal feed and coated on seeds to prevent blight and increase harvests.

In particular, chitosan is greatly favored as a diet food in the United States, and it has been registered on the list of natural food additives in Japan. Chitosan as a dietary ingredient hinders the absorption of cholesterol and lipids and aids in controlling hypertension. In general, cholesterol is mostly synthesized in the liver and is partially derived from food. It is a precursor of bile acid, passes through the duodenum, and sticks to the blood vessel walls, causing arteriosclerosis. Chitosan cations get dissolved in the acidic stomach and form strong ionic bonds with bile acid. They have an anion electric charge in the upper part of the small intestine and are discharged from the body, thereby reducing the blood concentration of cholesterol. In addition, chitosan cations weaken the activity of lipase, a lipid breakdown enzyme secreted from the pancreas, thereby preventing lipid degradation and absorption. Furthermore, the chitosan cations bind to the phosphate group sites on the droplet* surfaces in the duodenum, thereby hindering the action of lipase and reducing the absorption of fat. In addition, chitosan is known to discharge chlorine ions from the ingested salt, suppressing the activity of enzymes involved in hypertension and reducing blood pressure.

## 4.2 Chitosan oligosaccharides

### 4.2.1 Anticancer activity

Cancer has been known to be an incurable disease since the old times. Even more recently, the morbidity rate of cancer shows a continuously increasing trend. Although cancer diagnosis methods have advanced through the years, the vulnerability of people of all age groups to cancer has increased. Modern medicine has increased the life span of individuals, but the presence of water and other environmental pollutants due to modern civilization both directly and indirectly affect the human body.

In South Korea, the mortality rate associated with various types of cancers is 149 per 100,000 people per year and this rate has been increasing every year. Worldwide, the mortality rate of cancer is estimated to be approximately one million per year. In 2014, the Ministry of Health and Welfare announced statistical data analyzing the results of cancer patient enrollment. In the last 10 years, the mortality rate in South Korea has increased from 132.6 per 100,000 people in 2004 to 150.9 per 100,000 people in 2014 (13.8%). Of the various types of cancer, lung cancer shows the highest mortality rate (it increased from 27.3 in 2004 to 34.4 in 2014). In 2014, the mortality rate of liver cancer was 22.8, stomach cancer was 17.6, and colon cancer was 16.5, respectively. In addition, stomach cancer occurred most frequently in male patients (18.4%), followed by colon cancer (15.5%), and lung cancer (13.7%). The patients with one of these three types of cancers accounted for 47.6% of all the male cancer patients. Meanwhile, in the case of female cancer patients, thyroid cancer was the most frequent cancer found with a ratio of 35.8%, followed by breast cancer (15.6%) and colon cancer (9%), respectively. These three types of cancers accounted for 60% of all the female cancer patients.

The frequency of cancer onset generally increases with increasing age. In particular, skin cancer and prostate cancer occur mostly in elderly persons aged 70 years and are rarely found in persons aged <40 years. Uterine cancer develops in relatively young persons, and it is generally not found in persons aged ≥40 years. Liver cancer or digestive system cancers (for example, stomach cancer, colon cancer, and rectal cancer) occur more

---

* *Droplet*: A form of micelles, such as oil drops formed by lipids, which are fat-soluble, under water-soluble conditions in the body.

frequently in persons aged 40 to 59 years than in young persons. Among people aged ≤50 years, cancers occur more frequently in females, but in people aged >50 years, cancers occur more frequently in males.

Although leukemia can present in individuals of all ages, the incidence is high among South Korean people aged <30 years, according to the 2013 statistics. Hemangioma is a tumor that occurs most frequently in infants and children. Leukemia, malignant lymphoma, and cancers occurring in other hemopoietic organs account for 50% of cancers occurring in infants and children (2013 statistics of the causes of death, National Statistics Office). Therefore, cancers can occur in persons of all age groups. However, the possibility of developing cancer increases with increasing age, in general.

In South Korean males, the incidence of stomach cancer is the highest, followed by that of colon cancer and lung cancer, in order of precedence, whereas in South Korean females, the incidence of thyroid cancer is the highest, followed by that of breast cancer and colon cancer, in order of precedence. In the West, colon cancer occurs most frequently of all cancers in males, followed by lung cancer, whereas breast cancer occurs most frequently of all cancers in females, followed by lung cancer and liver cancer, in order of precedence. The higher incidence of stomach cancer in South Korean males as compared with in Western males can be attributed to the degree of consumption of boiled rice-centered meals, the frequent intake of salted foods, and the excessive intake of salt. The increasing rate of lung cancer is attributable to the population aging and an increase in the smoking population. The incidence of breast cancer and colon cancer is expected to increase in South Korea due to the increasing obese population and the consumption of a high-fat diet. In addition, pancreatic cancer and prostate cancer also appear to be closely related to environmental changes, such as the increase in environmental pollutants, and to lifestyle changes, such as increased alcohol consumption.

However, the question, *what is the identity of cancer?*, remains unanswered. Although the essence of cancer still cannot be accurately defined because the causes have not yet been identified, cancer can be said to be a cellular disease. A cell is the basic unit of all living organisms. The primary functions of the cells are cell division and proliferation. Normal cells follow a standard order for division and proliferation and such ability is rigorously controlled. However, when this order becomes broken for some reason, cells continue to divide infinitely; this abnormal cell growth eventually leads to death. Such diseases are defined as cancers. Although cancer cells originate from normal cells, the metabolic processes through which they ingest, degrade, and use nutrients are much more vigorous than those of normal cells because of their vigorous growth.

In addition, cancer cells can metastasize or infiltrate the surrounding areas. Infiltration is a process by which the number of cancer cells in a part of the body gradually increases and migrates to the nearby areas. These cancer cells continue to metastasize and destroy normal cells. This destructive action is continuous and irreversible, completely exhausting the individual. Metastasis is one of the reasons why cancer is incurable. Metastasis is a process by which a group of cancer cells in an organ infiltrate the surrounding tissues and spread to various regions in the body by entering the blood vessels or lymphatic vessels; they take root in other organs and tissues to start new proliferation. An abnormal lifestyle is a possible answer to the questions *why is cancer becoming a serious human disease?* and *why do certain cancers occur frequently in Koreans?* The present day lifestyles are thought to be the common way of living; however, they are the primary cause of cancer.

Although the causes of cancer are yet to be elucidated, assumptions can be made regarding which lifestyles increase the risk of cancers and which lifestyle modifications can reduce the risk. Therefore, the available knowledge on cancer can be used to lead a lifestyle that reduces the risk of cancer. Currently, more than half of cancer patients regain their healthy lives. According to the data from the Korea Central Cancer Registry, the five-year survival rate of domestic cancer patients has greatly increased in the last 20 years from 41.2% in 1993 to 1995 to 69.4% in 2009 to 2013. Although making lifestyle modifications is essential for an individual who has been completely cured of cancer, many people are negligent. According to experts, patients are not cautious and are unaware of the fact that primary/secondary metastasis can occur in new organs.

The risk of cancer relapse is four times higher in individuals with a history of cancer. This is because the genes of normal cells can be mutated due to poor lifestyle or the administration of radiation/anticancer treatment.

The types of secondary cancers can be predicted to some extent based on the type of primary cancer. The risk of colon cancer is 1.4 times higher in patients who have suffered from stomach cancer than in those who have not, while the risk of head and neck cancer is four times higher in those who have suffered from lung cancer as compared with those who have not. Even if patients have been completely cured of cancer, they should be regularly screened for six major cancers (stomach, large intestine, cervix, breast, liver, and lung cancers) and should regularly consume functional substances that can prevent cancers.

## 4.2.2   Anticancer activity by immunopotentiation

Cancer metastasis can be prevented by removing the source of cancer when cancer has been found at an early stage. In other cases, the life of the patient can be prolonged by the administration of anticancer drugs. Most anticancer drugs developed thus far are chemical substances and cause severe side effects because they do not selectively damage only cancer cells but also destroy normal cells. Therefore, treatment by immunotherapy is more desirable than treatment via the use of chemical substances, if possible. Immunotherapy is a method of directly activating those cells that are in charge of the immune system in our body to treat cancer or to enhance the effect of other treatments in treating cancer, reinforcing the immune system of the patient.

Immunity refers to the phenomenon where foreign substances (antigen) that invade the body are eliminated because they are engulfed and destroyed by white blood cells, macrophages, immune competent T-cells, and antibody-producing B-cells. White blood cells play a role in destroying relatively small foreign substances, such as bacteria. Macrophages are the cells that engulf relatively large foreign substances. The fragments (debris) formed after the destruction of the foreign substances by macrophages are discharged. Subsequently, immune competent cells form complexes with these fragments to determine whether the fragments are foreign substances and send signals to antibody-producing cells when attacks on these fragments are necessary. Upon receipt of these commands, the antibody-producing cells produce antibodies in large quantities that specifically react only to the foreign substances in order to remove them.

The intake of chitosan oligosaccharides may suppress cancers or prevent metastasis. Chitosan can activate macrophages or reinforce immune competent cells, thereby enabling antibody-producing cells to produce more antibodies to overcome cancer. In mouse models, chitosan is administered by intraperitoneal injections or subcutaneous injections rather than by oral administration in most cases. However, because chitosan is currently used as a dietary supplement and not as a drug, it should be administered orally. Chitosan is an insoluble macromolecule; therefore, it should be manufactured as oligosaccharides before it can be consumed to ensure that the effects are more clearly expressed.

Like Jeon and Kim (2002) reported, chitosan oligosaccharides with different molecular weights, such as oligosaccharide I (5–10 kDa), oligosaccharide II (1–5 kDa), and oligosaccharide III (<1 kDa), were manufactured. Specified amounts of chitosan oligosaccharides were administered every day into the abdominal cavities of rats transplanted with cervical cancer and melanoma* (sarcoma-180) tumor cells to examine the anticancer effects.

No significant changes were observed in the weight of the rats when 5 mg/kg of oligosaccharide I, oligosaccharide II, and oligosaccharide III each were administered for 24 days. However, higher tumor cell growth suppression rates were observed after treatment with oligosaccharide II, with 67% in ascites tumors and 74% in cervical cancer, in comparison with that with oligosaccharides I and oligosaccharides III. Therefore, the size of the oligosaccharides plays a very crucial role in their anticancer effects (Table 4.1).

---

* *Melanoma:* A tumor that mainly appears in the form of black spots on the skin as melanocytes turn into cancer cells.

Table 4.1 Effect of COSs on growth of implanted sarcoma 180 tumor cells and uterine cervix carcinoma tumor cells in mice

| Sample | Dosage (mg/kg/day) | Rat (head) | Melanoma (sarcoma-180 tumor cells) | | Cervical cancer (uterine cervix carcinoma tumor cells) | |
|---|---|---|---|---|---|---|
| | | | Tumor weight (mg) | Cancer suppression rate (%) | Tumor weight (mg) | Cancer suppression rate (%) |
| Control group | | 12 | 1032.5 ± 839.5 | — | 912.2 ± 612.1 | — |
| COS I (5 ~ 10 kDa) | 50 | 12 | 1147.0 ± 933.9 | — | 965.2 ± 839.7 | — |
| | 20 | 12 | 901.0 ± 741.7 | 12.7 | 803.3 ± 641.8 | 11.9 |
| | 10 | 12 | 795.5 ± 384.8 | 22.9 | 772.7 ± 592.2 | 15.3 |
| COS II (1 ~ 5 kDa) | 50 | 12 | 345.2 ± 218.6 | 66.6 | 240.5 ± 202.5 | 73.6 |
| | 20 | 12 | 665.6 ± 340.1 | 35.5 | 352.3 ± 331.1 | 61.4 |
| | 10 | 12 | 739.5 ± 351.8 | 28.4 | 669.5 ± 562.3 | 26.6 |
| COS III (<1 kDa) | 50 | 12 | 904.0 ± 510.3 | 12.4 | 665.0 ± 477.9 | 27.1 |
| | 20 | 12 | 874.5 ± 516.6 | 15.3 | 841.1 ± 602.1 | 7.8 |
| | 10 | 12 | 973.5 ± 417.1 | 5.7 | 879.9 ± 650.3 | 3.5 |

COS: Chitosan oligosaccharides.

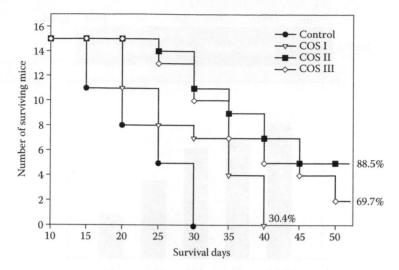

*Figure 4.1* Effects of chitosan oligosaccharide treatment on the survival of rats transplanted with melanoma cells.

Figure 4.1 shows the anticancer effects of chitosan oligosaccharide treatment in rats transplanted with melanoma tumor cells. The rats transplanted with melanoma cancer cells that were not treated died within 30 days, while approximately 89% of the rats transplanted with melanoma cancer cells that were treated with chitosan oligosaccharides (molecular weight: 3 ~ 5 kDa) survived even after 50 days, indicating that chitosan oligosaccharides have anticancer effects.

Our bodies consist of cells and matrix (the substance that fills the space between the cells). The main components of the matrix are proteins, and carbohydrates also play a role in filling the spaces between the cells. In the term *matrix metalloproteinase* (MMP), the word *metallo* signifies a metal component such as zinc and manganese, and the word *proteinase* indicates an enzyme that degrades proteins. Therefore, MMPs refer to the enzymes that contain metal components in their chemical structures and dissolve the matrix proteins. MMPs widely exist in the tissues and cells of microorganisms, animals, and plants. MMPs are involved not only in normal biological processes, such as embryogeny, implantation, organogenesis, nerve growth, ovulation, uterine expansion, embryogenesis, wound healing, angiogenesis, and apoptosis, but also in the diverse pathological processes of diseases such as arthritis, cancer, wrinkling, cardiovascular diseases, neurogenic diseases, gastric ulcer, and chronic inflammations.

In particular, MMP-9 plays an important role in cancer metastasis; therefore, the MMP-9 activity inhibitory effects of chitosan oligosaccharides were reviewed in this study. According to the study results reported

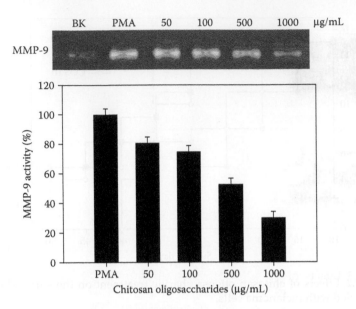

*Figure 4.2* MMP-9 activity inhibitory effects of chitosan oligosaccharides in human skin cells; PMA: phorbol 12-myristate 13-acetate.

by Kim and Kim (2006), MMP-9 activity was dose-dependently suppressed by chitosan oligosaccharides at the concentrations shown in Figure 4.2.

Furthermore, when liver cancer cells were treated with chitosan oligosaccharides for 72 h, apoptosis was induced with increasing chitosan oligosaccharide concentration, leading to the extinction of cancer cells. Liver cancer cells was damaged by chitosan oligosaccharides dose-dependently (Figure 4.3). Since chitosan oligosaccharides inhibit cancer metastasis and destroy cancer cells, they are useful in cancer treatment and aid in the prevention of cancers. They can be used as functional food materials.

## 4.2.3   Prevention of weight loss due to cancer

In general, body weight sharply decreases during cancer, and this may be prevented by chitosan oligosaccharides. A study conducted by Professor Okuda (1994) concluded that cancer causes weight loss in rats. He injected melanoma (sarcoma-180) cells into the abdominal cavities of rats and examined changes in their body fat. The rats' body fat was shown to remarkably decrease in those transplanted with cancer cells, and the cause was thought to be a loss of appetite.

However, the results of the study indicated that cancer cells secrete substances that degrade neutral fat stored in fat cells (Table 4.2). When the fat

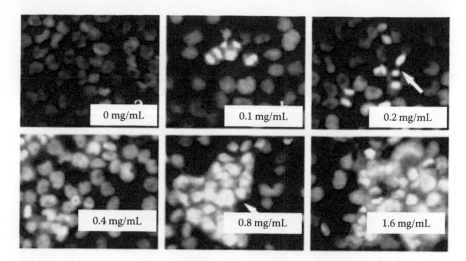

*Figure 4.3* Effects of chitosan oligosaccharides on human liver cancer cells (SMMC-7721).

*Table 4.2* Lipolysis activity of toxohormone-L in the ascites of various cancers

| Ascites | | Lipolysis activity (mg/protein) |
|---|---|---|
| Cancerous ascites | Melanoma (sarcoma-180) (rat) | $2.7 \pm 0.3$ |
| | Liver cancer (human) | $7.2 \pm 1.7$ |
| | Lung cancer (human) | $7.7 \pm 1.0$ |
| | Malignant ovarian tumor (human) | $7.3 \pm 0.3$ |
| Noncancerous ascites | Peritonitis (rat) | 0 |
| | Liver cirrhosis (human) | 0 |

stored in the fat cells decreases, it is degraded into fatty acid and glycerol, which is used in energy production. In addition, cancer cells in the abdominal cavity lead to ascites, where toxohormone-L (a toxic substance extracted from cancer cells that inhibits catalase activity) degrades the fat secreted from cancer cells. Although toxohormone-L is present in the ascites of rats transplanted with melanoma (sarcoma-180), human liver cancer ascites, human lung cancer pleural fluid, and malignant ovarian tumor ascites, the activity of toxohormone-L is not exhibited in ascites of non-cancer diseases, such as rat peritonitis and human hepatic cirrhosis (Table 4.2).

Although toxohormone-L is generally present in ascites without cancer activity, the concentration of toxohormone-L is less and the concentrations of substances that inhibit the toxohormone-L activity are more in such ascites; therefore, the fat-degrading activity of toxohormone-L is absent. Furthermore, toxohormone-L was isolated and purified from human liver

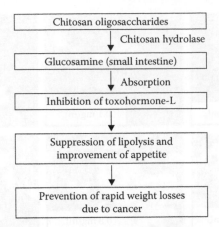

*Figure 4.4* Weight loss-preventing effect of chitosan oligosaccharides.

cancer ascites in a study reported by Okhuda (1994), and the results indicated that toxohormone-L not only degrades fat but also reduces appetite. Toxohormone-L is a glycoprotein with a molecular weight of approximately 70,000 kDa and contains aspartic acid at its N-terminal. When 7.2 and 14.4 µg of purified toxohormone-L were injected into the lateral ventricles of rats, a larger decline in the appetite of the rats injected with 14.4 µg of purified toxohormone-L was observed in comparison with the appetite of those injected with 7.2 µg of purified toxohormone-L.

In other words, one of the causes of the rapid weight loss seen in cancer patients is the appetite decline that occurs as soon as fat is degraded by the toxohormone-L secreted from cancer cells. Toxohormone-L also decreases these individuals' appetite by exciting the satiety center. Although chitosan alone cannot inhibit the action of toxohormone-L, glucosamine, which is a degradation product of chitosan, it has been shown to inhibit the action of toxohormone-L. However, acetyl glucosamine, which is a degradation product of chitin, does not show this inhibitory action. The glucosamine produced by the degradation of chitosan in the gut inhibits the toxohormone-L secreted from cancer cells, thereby inhibiting lipolysis and preventing rapid weight loss (Figure 4.4).

## 4.2.4   Anti-aging

Most living organisms on the Earth maintain their life using the energy obtained from food, oxidizing it with the oxygen in the air. Reactive oxygen species* are dangerous to the living body tissues, as they lead to

---

* Oxygen in the state of energy that has rich reactivity unlike stable oxygen, which has a defensive mechanism that shows characteristics to human bodies to decompose substances.

oxidization and damage cells. Furthermore, reactive oxygen compounds such as hyperoxide ($O_2^-$) and hydrogen peroxide ($H_2O_2$) are produced in large quantities even in biodefense processes intended to remove pathogens or foreign substances by their strong germicidal actions designed to protect the human body from pathogens.

Antioxidation means the inhibition of oxidation. It is a concept that appears mainly when explaining the cell aging process and the prevention of cell aging. Cell aging means the oxidation of the cells. Oxygen that enters the body through breathing is beneficial to the body, but reactive oxygen species are also produced by this process. Reactive oxygen is in an unstable state, which adversely affects animal bodies. In other words, removing active oxygen is the key to preventing cell oxidation and cell aging.

Reactive oxygen species damage cells or cell organelles and oxidize the amino acids of various proteins in the living body, leading to the degradation of protein functions. This also causes damage to nucleic acids and may prompt nucleic acid base deformation, nucleic acid base liberation, bond cleavage, or oxidative degradation of sugars, leading to mutations or cancers. Therefore, the generation of reactive oxygen should be minimized. Smoking, which massively produces reactive oxygen, must be avoided and exposure to various harmful environments such as pollution, ultraviolet rays, and food additives should be minimized. Stress should be relieved appropriately within a short time so that it will not build up. Appropriate but not excessive exercise is also necessary. Taking antioxidants can also prevent the production of active oxygen in the body. Eating fresh vegetables and fruits that are rich in vitamins and minerals is good and drinking green or black tea instead of coffee is a sound practice. However, as people age, more reactive oxygen species are produced and the antioxidative ability in the body gradually declines, leading to a reduction in the elimination of reactive oxygen species from the body by only eating vegetables or fruits. In this case, one must consume vitamin E (tocopherol), vitamin C, beta-carotene (β-carotene), selenium, melatonin,* and propolis, which are strong antioxidative compounds.

Since the beginning of the twentieth century, the average life span of humans has been continuously increasing, primarily in advanced countries. It has been found that the average life span in the 1990s was 66% longer in males and 71% longer in females in comparison with that in the 1900s, indicating that the proportion of elderly in the population has been rapidly increasing. In South Korea, the population aged ≥65 years was 3.74% in the 1960s and 3.87% in the 1980s, respectively; it subsequently increased to 6.35% in the 2000s and is expected to be 11.45% in 2020.

---

* *Melatonin*: A hormone secreted from the pineal gland, which controls biorhythms and performs actions such as anti-aging, vigor promotion, and the inhibition of diseases such as cancers.

Worldwide, the proportion of elderly in the population was 5.1% in 1960, 5.7% in 1980, and 6.6% in 2000; this is expected to become 8.1% in 2020. This increase in the average life span is attributed to decreased infant mortality rates in the early years. However, since the average life span is increasing even in recent years and the decreases in infant birth rates and mortality rates have been stagnant, the increase in the average life span should also be attributed to the removal of causes of death in elderly persons in addition to decreases in their mortality rates. Common causes of death in elderly persons include heart diseases, cancer, and diabetes. Since these diseases have been conquered to some extent, the causes of death in elderly persons have decreased, leading to increased life span.

The life spans of all living organisms are finite, and the maximum life span varies among species. The maximum life span ranges from three years in the case of rodents to more than 100 years in the case of primates. The maximum life span of humans is estimated to be approximately 150 years. However, answers to questions such as *what are the determinants of the life spans as such?*, *why the life spans of a living organism are finite?*, and *why the life spans are different among species?* are still debatable. In general, after animals have become mature, all their physical functions gradually decrease until they eventually die. If this stage in which physical functions decrease is regarded to be aging, aging can be said to be an inevitable stage that must be participated in before natural death occurs.

The definition of aging is also interpreted in various ways, with some scholars regarding aging as simply getting old, while others suggesting the decline in physical functions that appears in animals to be aging. Some scholars also consider the last stage of growth and development that begins from the stage of fertilization as aging. However, one thing in common across the board is that aging is interpreted as a stage detrimental to individuals, which eventually leads to death. The mechanism of aging has not yet been clearly elucidated, but all organs show changes in their structures and degeneration of their functions as they get old. As a result, changes in the body appear in all aspects including anatomical, biochemical, physiological, and behavioral aspects. The functions of all organs decline as they get old and these functional changes occur independently. However, the decline in the functions of each organ eventually leads to declines in the entire physical function of the body. In addition, the aging of higher organs such as the brain and thymus promote aging of other organs regulated by these organs. The decline in the immune system due to aging reduces resistance to various diseases and external stresses. The cause of this decline in immune functions can be regarded to be the decline in the functions of immune competent cells due to the degeneration of the thymus.

If the immune system is compromised, the degeneration of all internal organs will begin and this change can be regarded as aging. In other words, as aging begins, physical functions, the adaptability to changes in the environment, the ability to control various external and internal stresses, and the defense capability of hosts declines and susceptibility to pathological conditions increases. Therefore, living bodies become susceptible to various diseases with aging and their life spans can be determined by the kinds and degrees of such diseases.

The progression of aging depends largely on two elements, a species-specific genetic component and the interactions between surrounding environments and these genetic components. Aging is affected by genetic backgrounds, lifestyles, and nutrition factors. However, some of these aging-promoting factors can be prevented or controlled. For example, noninsulin-dependent diabetes accelerates aging. However, noninsulin-dependent diabetes can be prevented by weight control or diet therapy and normal conditions be recovered even after contracting the disease. Therefore, the disease can be prevented by controlling the lifestyle or dietary intake, thereby delaying the progression of aging. Hence, a varying degree of aging is largely observed among individuals.

This hypothesis states that the free radicals generated in the normal metabolic process in the living body react with biomolecules to damage the cells, and that the generation of free radicals increases with age, leading to gradual declines in cell functions that eventually result in the phenomenon of aging. This hypothesis was argued by Harman in 1956, who indicated that free radicals act on cells and connective tissues to produce harmful substances; the accumulation of these harmful substances is a fundamental cause of aging and chronic degenerative diseases.

Free radicals refer to atoms or molecules having unpaired electrons. Oxygen is essential for the production of energy necessary for living bodies. One oxygen molecule inhaled into the body gets converted into two molecules of water ($H_2O$), which is a stable reducing substance when it has received four electrons. However, when it receives only one electron for some reason, a superoxide anion radical ($O_2^-$) is generated. In cells, superoxide anion radicals are generated by the reactions of enzymes such as xanthine oxidase, cytochrome P-450, and aldehyde oxidase; these superoxide anion radicals can get easily converted into hydrogen peroxide ($H_2O_2$) by superoxide dismutase (SOD).[*] The superoxide anion radicals and $H_2O_2$ together form hydroxyl radicals ($\bullet$ OH$^-$) in reactions mediated by iron (Fe). A hydroxyl radical is a highly reactive oxidant that reacts with adjacent macromolecule substances to form another radical. This reaction occurs sequentially until the free radical meets another radical and forms an electron pair, or until it reacts with an antioxidant.

---

[*] *Superoxide dismutase*: An enzyme that catalyzes the disproportionation reactions ($2O_2^- \cdot + 2H+ \rightarrow O_2 + H_2O_2$) of superoxide ion radicals ($O_2^- \cdot$)

In the living body, oxygen is reduced by various mechanisms and converted into superoxide anion radicals; a representative example of such reactions occurs in the mitochondria.* Approximately 95% of the oxygen inhaled by us is used in the energy metabolism of mitochondria and 95% of the oxygen used gets converted to water through the respiratory chain of the mitochondria. However, some oxygen (approximately 3% to 5% of the oxygen used in the mitochondria) pair with leaking electrons from the respiratory chain and is reduced into superoxide anion radicals.

As such, free radicals are generated in the normal cell metabolic process, and their generation is increased by environmental factors such as radiation, drugs, and ozone. Macromolecule substances in the living body that react with free radicals include unsaturated fatty acids, proteins, and deoxyribonucleic acid (DNA). Free radicals interact with unsaturated fatty acids to form lipid peroxides, which react with amino groups such as proteins and nucleic acids to form lipofuscin, which is a fluorescent substance. Lipofuscin is often known as senile plaques. In addition, since the reaction with unsaturated fatty acids occurs sequentially to continuously induce the formation of many free radicals, the oxidation of unsaturated fatty acids is considered to be the most important reaction among free radical-forming reactions occurring in the cells. Since unsaturated fatty acids are abundantly contained in cell membranes, this action of free radicals not only causes damage to cell membranes but also deforms the structures of cell membranes or the microstructural membranes of cells, such as the mitochondria or ribosomes, when free radicals have been accumulated, damaging the travel or functions of substances and resulting in aging.

The byproducts resulting from the reactions between free radicals and body proteins are an important cause of aging: in other words, the reactants bound to the proteins generated in the processes of the oxidation and reduction of body proteins and the substances generated by active sequential reactions of such substances lead to aging and various diseases. Such examples include the accumulation of lipofuscin and aldehyde-protein adducts at regions at which arteries have been hardened. As animals get old, the DNA activity decreases while the cross-linking between the two strands of chains increases. When free radicals react with DNA molecules, the reduction of the activity of the DNA molecules is accelerated and inadequate gene expression is caused, damaging physical functions. Consequently, free radicals increase the cross-linking of connective tissues, damage cell membranes, and induce DNA mutations, thereby impairing the functions of body proteins. The results of these free radical reactions can be said to be accumulated in the body

---

* *Mitochondria*: A rod component present in the cytoplasm of cells that is a major site of energy production through the degradation of foods.

over time, leading to the progression of aging. To minimize damage by free radicals, superoxide anion radicals and $H_2O_2$ should be removed as soon as they are formed in the metabolic process. Cells are equipped with defense systems such as compartmentalization and antioxidation to protect themselves from free radicals. The antioxidative substances include enzymes generated in cells, such as glutathione peroxidase (GSH-PX)[*] superoxide dismutase enzyme (SOD), and catalase;[†] and nutrients and metabolites supplied from the outside of cells such as vitamin A, vitamin C, vitamin E, and carotene.

It is important to maintain the appropriate concentrations of these antioxidants in the cells because they play an important role in inhibiting the accumulation of free radicals in the body. The theories that explain the process by which free radicals generated during the metabolic process are involved in aging have emerged as several distinct hypotheses based on the various viewpoints. However, the core theory is that if genetic information is repeatedly used, it will be exhausted and will lead to aging, much like how machines that are continuously used become worn out. Genetic information is consumed because free radicals gradually destroy cells and enzymes and the living body exhausts normal cells and enzymes, resulting in aging and death.

## 4.2.5   Chitosan oligosaccharides' free radical scavenging activity

Chitosan oligosaccharides inhibit the accumulation of free radicals. Chitosan oligosaccharides (molecular weights ≤1,000 kDa and 1,000–3,000 kDa) produced by decomposing chitosan using enzymes were studied for radical scavenging activity. The experimental group showed higher radical scavenging activity for the hydroxyl radicals, superoxide radicals, and alkyl radicals in comparison with the control group without the addition of any chitosan oligosaccharide.[‡] The chitosan oligosaccharides that had molecular weights ≤1,000 kDa showed higher radical scavenging activity (Figure 4.5). When the radical scavenging activity levels of chitosan oligosaccharides with molecular weights ≤1,000 kDa were examined according to their concentrations, most of the chitosan oligosaccharides showed radical scavenging activity levels of at least 95% in cases in which their concentration was at least 0.05% (Figure 4.6).

The free radical theory, which is the most highly supported aging theory, states that cells are gradually damaged by the free radicals with

---

[*] *Glutathione peroxidase (GSH-Px)*: An enzyme that catalyzes the reactions that generate oxidized glutathione and water or alcohol from glutathione and hydrogen peroxides or lipid peroxides.

[†] *Catalase*: An enzyme that catalyzes the reactions that degrade hydrogen peroxides.

[‡] *Control group*: A group that was set as the criterion when two or more subjects were compared with each other.

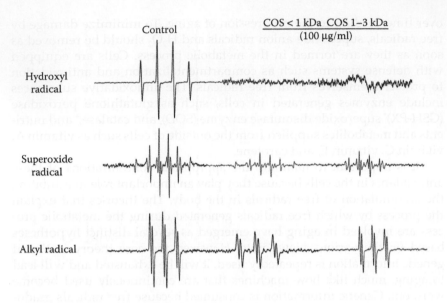

***Figure 4.5*** Chitosan oligosaccharides' radical scavenging activity effects obtained using electron spin resonance.

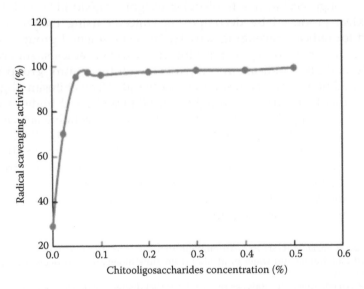

***Figure 4.6*** Radical scavenging activity of chitosan oligosaccharides' according to their concentrations.

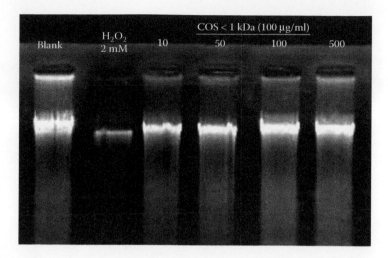

*Figure 4.7* Effects of chitosan oligosaccharides to DNA damage inhibition by hydrogen peroxides.

strong reactivity, which are generated continuously, and that the accumulation of such damage leads to declines in cellular functions. However, as shown in Figure 4.7, although DNA molecules were damaged by $H_2O_2$, when treated with chitosan oligosaccharides, the damage to these molecules was inhibited in a concentration-dependent manner. The intake of chitosan oligosaccharides can reduce the generation of free radicals in living bodies, preventing and treating adult diseases caused by aging and free radicals such as cancers, declines in immunity, and arteriosclerosis.

# chapter five

# Physiological functions of glucosamine

## 5.1 Promotion of appetite

Chitosan is decomposed into glucosamine by the action of chitosanase or lysozyme,* and glucosamine promotes appetite. In this context, at first, we explain the phenomenon of appetite. At that time, gold therapy was performed on patients with rheumatism. Gold therapy is a method of treatment in which patients drink a substance made of glucose particles coated with gold. However, surprisingly, patients treated with gold therapy began to gain weight. When the brain of a dead patient with rheumatism was accidentally examined, it was observed that some of the cell groups of the hypothalamus in the brain were destroyed.

In an experimental setup by Anand et al. (1951), the region called the ventromedial hypothalamus in the hypothalamus of 30 monkeys was destroyed, and all but one became obese. Generally, when animals have eaten to some extent, they stop eating, as they feel satiated. However, animals do not feel satiated when the ventromedial hypothalamus is damaged or destroyed. The findings of this study revealed the ventromedial hypothalamus in the hypothalamus to be a part of the brain that enables the feeling of satiety, called the satiety center nerve. Following 10 years of examination of the satiety center, a feeding center was discovered. An experiment was carried out to disrupt the satiety center in a cat by Professors Brobeck and Anand of Yale University in the United States. In the skull, a small hole was made to insert a needle electrode and an electrical current was administered to burn off the satiety center. However, when the satiety center was damaged, the cat started to gain flesh rather than losing it. An investigation on the cat was conducted in detail as the results obtained were found to be strange. Ultimately, it was observed that a region located laterally 1 mm away from the satiety center was also destroyed, which caused the cat to refuse the food. The destroyed region

---

* *Lysozyme*: An enzyme that degrades the cell walls of bacteria, which is present in egg fluid, body fluid, tears, and white blood cells.

was the hypothalamus lateral nucleus and the center that led the cat to feel hunger is known as the feeding center.

The satiety center was destroyed due to the substance made by coating gold on glucose. It was observed that glucose has an affinity to accumulate at the satiety center, so the glucose in this particular substance was present largely at the satiety center of it and surrounded by gold. The increased blood sugar levels that occur after eating stimulates the satiety center, which causes satiety and led the cat to stop eating.

The fact that glucose stimulates the satiety center gave an idea to Professor Sakada and colleagues from the School of Medicine, Oita University in Japan that glucosamine, which is a chitosan hydrolysate, could also enhance appetite. Thus, they investigated the effects of various sugars on appetite. It was found that oral administration of an aqueous solution of glucosamine in rats resulted in increased appetite. Consequently, the rats ate more food and when the vagus nerve,* which is located between the liver and the diaphragm, was cut, no increase was noted in appetite. This occurred due to the fact that the glucosamine absorbed from the gut enters the liver through the portal vein (the capillary plexus formed because the veins returning to the heart blocked branches) while stimulating the vagus nerves distributed in the liver, and this stimulus ultimately reaches the feeding center, resulting in appetite.

The stimulus from the periphery, such as the liver, can also reach the feeding center as it also dominates the vagus nerves. Therefore, the intake of glucosamine, a degradation product of chitosan oligosaccharides, can improve the loss of appetite.

## 5.2   Arthritis treatment

There are two types of arthritis: inflammatory arthritis and noninflammatory arthritis. Though inflammatory arthritis is often misunderstood as the inflammation of the joint caused by the invasion of bacteria, it is, in fact, an inflammatory response exerted by leukocytes, antibodies, or complements,† which are present in the joints. The frequently occurring inflammatory arthritis is rheumatoid arthritis and the most representative noninflammatory arthritis is osteoarthritis, which is also the most

---

* *Vagus nerve*: One of the cranial nerves, specifically the tenth cranial nerve. It consists of motor nerves (larynx), sensory nerves (larynx, visceral), and autonomic nerves (parasympathetic nerves). Vagus nerve activities cause bronchoconstriction, the inhibition of cardiac activities, the promotion of the movements of digestive tracts, and the acceleration of parasympathetic nerves such as the promotion of secretion of digestive juices.
† *Complement*: Protein substances in the fresh serum of normal animals. It possesses bactericidal properties and is involved in immune responses.

representative of all types of arthritis. Arthritis caused by the invasion of bacteria is called purulent arthritis and the one caused by the invasion of the virus is called viral arthritis. Osteoarthritis is generally called degenerative arthritis as it naturally occurs as humans age. Degenerative arthritis occurs mainly in the late forties, though 70% of individuals aged 65 years or more suffer from this disease, and most individuals aged 75 years or more have this disease. There are 68 joints in the human body, which play different roles in supporting and moving the body. Each joint consists of bones around the cartilage and a membrane surrounding the joint. The cartilage primarily serves for moisturizing, is elastic, and plays the role of a buffer between bones.

OA, which is the most common form of arthritis, affects the articular cartilage that is a greenish-white, shiny, and slippery substance attached to the distal end of the bone. It also affects the cartilages and bones around and inside the joints (the subchondral bones, the ends of the bones connected to the cartilages); the films around the joints; and the muscles attached to the joints besides the articular cartilage. As osteoarthritis progresses, the cartilages of the joints dry up and, as a result, they fail to absorb shocks between the bones. When the disease progresses further, the bones receive stimuli and become abnormally hardened (eburnation), and pockets full of liquid (cartilage and cysts) may form in the bones. Evidently, as the cartilage deteriorates, the bones directly produce friction, the pain becomes more severe, the bones are deformed, and, eventually, inflammation is induced. In severe cases, the cartilage is completely decayed so that both ends of the bones are completely exposed. Drug therapy should be applied to test osteoarthritis for long periods of time along with rest and exercise.

Rheumatoid arthritis is a chronic multi-organ disease of unknown etiology. It is characterized by symmetrical chronic inflammatory synovitis (the inflammation of the membrane wrapping the joint) occurring in joints on both sides (primarily the hands, wrists, feet, and ankles). This arthritis shows diverse progress, and most patients undergo processes in which the aggravation and relief of the disease are repeated and, to some extent, also experience hindrance to a normal life. Rheumatoid arthritis occurs in all races all around the world and its prevalence (the rate people having this disease for a period of one year in the entire population) is reported to be approximately 0.3% to 2.1% and 0.8% globally and in the Asian region, respectively. This disease progresses most frequently in the thirties and forties and occurs three times more frequently among females than among males.

As the names of osteoarthritis and rheumatoid arthritis are similar and both cause joint pain, they are often confused. However, they are different diseases. Rheumatoid arthritis affects the immune system. The characteristics that distinguish them are presented in Table 5.1.

***Table 5.1*** Characteristics to distinguish osteoarthritis and rheumatoid
arthritis from each other

| Osteoarthritis | Rheumatoid arthritis |
| --- | --- |
| Normally occurs after the age of 40 years | Initially, occurs at an age between 25 and 50 years |
| Gradually progresses over several years | Frequently occurs without warning and disappears |
| Generally begins involving only the joints on one side of the body | Generally appears simultaneously on both sides of the body (e.g., both hands) |
| Symptoms such as red spots, fever, and inflammations are rare | Symptoms such as red spots, fever, and inflammations are common |
| Primarily affects the knee, the hand, the buttocks, the feet, the waist, and the joints. Rarely occurs in the finger joints, the wrist, or the shoulder | Affects not only the finger joint, the wrist, the elbow, and the shoulder but also almost all joints |
| Does not cause overall subjective symptoms of the disease | Causes overall subjective symptoms of weight loss, diseases accompanied by fever, and fatigue |

## 5.3   *General misunderstanding of osteoarthritis*

The onset of osteoarthritis generally occurs with aging; however, it can be prevented through appropriate exercise. Since secondary osteoarthritis caused by damage or repetitive shocks may be attributable to both using and not using the joints, unlike with respect to primary osteoarthritis, it is not caused by wear due to excessive motions or exercise and damage. Currently, drug therapy and surgery are the primary methods of treatment for osteoarthritis. Though both acetaminophen and nonsteroidal anti-inflammatory drugs (NSAIDs),* which are primarily used in drug therapy, are widely employed as effective analgesics and anti-inflammatory drugs, it has been revealed that their administration may further aggravate osteoarthritis in the long term, as they cause secondary side-effects, such as gastrointestinal disorder, when taken for a long time, and they do not fundamentally treat osteoarthritis but instead just relieve pain and inflammation. In addition, in the case of surgery, there is a risk of death or becoming disabled even when the surgery has been successful and, as the life span of artificial joints is generally 10 to 15 years, additional surgery is typically required.

* *Nonsteroidal anti-inflammatories (NSAIDs)*: Substances that alleviate pain while removing inflammations.

### 5.3.1 New hope for arthritis treatment

In the 2004 book *Arthritis Treatment Method*, Jason Theodosakis, MD, introduces an osteoarthritis treatment method by using glucosamine, chondroitin sulfuric acid, vitamin C, and manganese. In the clinical results, he disclosed that the effects of this method begin to appear in two to three weeks of treating osteoarthritis, then more so in four to eight weeks, and finally with at least 90% of effects visible in six months at the latest. Glucosamine is an important part of chitosan and primarily constitutes the structures of bones, cartilage, skin, nails, hair, and other body tissues. Glucosamine performs the same actions when taken in food. Glucosamine shows the following two actions: it binds well to hydrophilic molecules* and stimulates cartilage cells to make more collagen and proteoglycan, and normalizes the cartilage metabolic process to prevent the destruction of cartilage.

Most of the glucosamine products that are currently available in South Korea are made by decomposing chitosan using hydrochloric acid. As glucosamine is made by decomposing by hydrochloric acid, the products are known as glucosamine hydrochloric acid (glucosamine HCl). A 100% enzymatically decomposed glucosamine production process that decomposes chitosan oligosaccharides has been developed, and this technology has been transferred to an enterprise that is now producing the only enzyme-decomposed glucosamine in the world.

## 5.4 Shoulder discomfort and low back pain relieving effects

### 5.4.1 Stimulation of parasympathetic nerves and arterioles

It is important to note that glucosamine, which is a degradation product of chitosan oligosaccharides, stimulates the vagus nerves distributed in the liver to excite the feeding center, as the feeding center is not only the center for developing hunger sensation but can also be considered as a center of the parasympathetic nerves. Therefore, the stimulation of the vagus nerve by the glucosamine may possibly reach the feeding center, exciting the parasympathetic nerves and transmitting the excitation to the whole body.

The noradrenalin† that is secreted from the periphery of the sympathetic nerves generally causes the contraction of arterioles to induce a blood circulation disturbance at the periphery. On the contrary, acetylcholine secreted from the parasympathetic nerves dilates the arterioles to

---

* *Proteoglycan*: A generic term for molecule groups in which proteins are bound to the side chain of a sugar named glycosaminoglycan.
† *Noradrenaline*: A type of catecholamine hormone secreted from the adrenal medulla, which is also called norepinephrine. Its biological activity is similar to that of adrenaline but lower than that of adrenaline.

improve peripheral circulations. Evidently, acetylcholine is secreted not only from the parasympathetic nerves but also from the nerves that do not belong to the category of sympathetic nerves.

When acetylcholine acts on the endothelial cells located inside the arterioles, the reactions (catalyzed by nitric oxide synthase), which produce nitrogen monoxide (NO) from arginine, are promoted so that the arterioles are dilated (Figure 5.1).

A possibility that the glucosamine generated by the degradation of chitosan oligosaccharides stimulates the *afferent nerve** in the vagus nerve and the autonomic nerve (parasympathetic nerve) center and intervenes in the process of dilating the arterioles to improve the peripheral circulation was found. Though the peripheral circulation belongs to the circulatory system in a broad sense, the heart and the aorta have been considered important, as the main circulatory organs and the peripheral circulation has been relatively undervalued.

Round cross-sections of the arteriole and the capillary vessel are presented in Figure 5.2. The arteries that come out from the heart reach the arterioles via the aorta and middle arteries. As smooth muscle cells are located in the middle (between the outer membrane and endothelial cells), these arteries can contract and relax by themselves. However, as capillary vessels have no smooth muscle cells, they cannot contract or relax.

The capillary vessels are passively contracted or dilated by changes in the volume of blood resulting from the contraction and dilatation of the arterioles by noradrenaline and acetylcholine (choline acetylide, which is

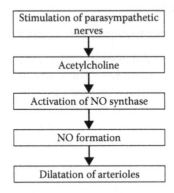

*Figure 5.1* The stimulation of parasympathetic nerves and the dilatation of arterioles.

* *Afferent nerve*: The nervous system is largely divided into the central nervous system (brain and spinal cord) and the peripheral nervous system, and the peripheral nervous system includes afferent and efferent nerves. The nerves that transmit information from receptors responding to changes in the outside world or in the living body to the central nervous system are called afferent nerves.

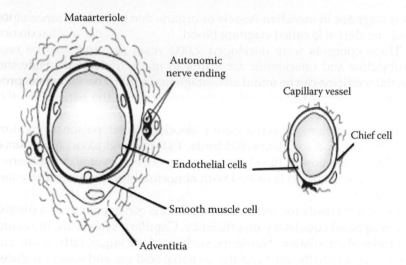

*Figure 5.2* Arterioles and capillary vessels.

a neurotransmitter) secreted from the autonomic nerve endings distributed in the arterioles.

The capillary vessels supply oxygen, blood sugar, and fatty acids in the blood to the cells. Carbon dioxide ($CO_2$) and water ($H_2O$) discharged by the cells is transported. Carbon dioxide gas is discharged by respiration and water is discharged through urination.

The capillary vessels, which are directly and closely related with the cell metabolism, play an important role in the circulatory system along with the heart, though the peripheral circulation around the capillary vessels has not been considered in modern medicine.

## 5.4.2   Peripheral circulation in oriental medicine

The peripheral circulation has been considered to be an important concept in Oriental medicine. The concept of extravasated blood or water poison[*] is related with the peripheral circulation.

Chinese medicine uses the term extravasated blood, which refers to a disease symptom developed when the blood in the body does not circulate at a certain location and is divided into vitiated blood and stagnant blood. Vitiated blood overflows from the meridian, is stagnant in the spaces between tissues, and is degraded. On the other hand, the blood

---

[*] *Water poison:* In the body, not only is water that is beneficial to the body present, but also bad water is generated by itself when body conditions are not good or for other reasons. Such bad water is called water poison.

that is stagnant in meridian vessels or organs due to the hindrance of the blood circulation is called stagnant blood.

These concepts were developed 2,000 years ago and may be seen as subjective and unscientific according to modern medicine. However, Oriental medicine can be found advantageous in that it considers patients' pain and thereby examines the entire condition of the patient so as to judge their disease.

The applications of extravasated blood or water poison to modern medicine can lead to unexpected hints. Extravasated blood is a disease that hinders the flow of blood among energy/blood/water.* It is reported that extravasated blood is related with abnormalities in energy and water in many cases.

In modern medicine, extravasated blood is considered to be a disease with peripheral circulatory insufficiency. Capillary vessels are the center of peripheral circulation. Nutrients, such as blood sugar, fatty acids, and oxygen, are sent to the cells and the carbonic acid gas and water produced by the cells are transported through capillary vessels. In addition, cells outside of blood vessels such as muscle cells or fat cells are not directly surrounded by blood but are contained in cell interstitial fluid that exudes from the capillary vessels.

### 5.4.3   Shoulder discomfort and low back pain caused by peripheral circulatory insufficiency

The extravasated blood becomes cold and the supply of nutrients and oxygen to the muscle cells become insufficient, causing shoulder discomfort or low back pain, when the temperature of the body surface is lowered due to peripheral circulatory insufficiency. The muscles are considered to be organs that repeat the movements of contraction and relaxation, and the act of muscle contraction causes shoulder discomfort or the low back pain stemming from the muscles.

---

* *Energy/blood/water*: This is a term of Oriental medicine that refers to the energy source that supplies energy to the internal organs. In the classical theory of Oriental medicine, the internal organs of the human body include six viscera and the six entrails or six parts, which are maintained with the circulation of qi and blood that circulates in the body at a certain rhythm. The internal organs of the human body comprise five viscera and the six entrail parts. Specifically, there are the five viscera of the liver, the heart, the spleen, the lungs, and the kidneys; and the six entrails of the gall bladder, the stomach, the small intestine, the three parts of the body (the body is divided into the upper part, middle part, and lower part), and the bladder. In Oriental medicine, the heart sack (the invisible component that performs the functions of the heart on behalf of the heart) is added to the five viscera and it is reported that there are instead six viscera. The meridian system is the circulation path of these qi and blood, and it is reported that qi circulates outside the meridians and that blood circulates in the meridians.

When the calcium ions ($Ca^{2+}$) contained in the sarcoplasmic reticulum*
come out and gather around the myosin proteins and actin fiber proteins
to narrow the spaces among the actin fiber proteins, muscle contraction
occurs. If muscle contraction is maintained for a long time, the shoulders
become stiffened or muscle pain occurs. The calcium ions that come out
from the sarcoplasmic reticulum must be re-accommodated by the sarcoplasmic reticulum so that the state of muscle contraction is changed
into the state of muscle relaxation. However, the adenosine triphospha-
tase present on the membranes of the sarcoplasmic reticulum degrades
the energy-accumulating substance, and the resultant energy enables the
calcium ions to enter the sarcoplasmic reticulum (Figure 5.3); thus, the
accommodation of calcium ions requires energy.

When sugar or fatty acids ingested by humans are oxidized in muscle
cells, energy is produced. The blood does not flow to the capillary vessels,
stopping the supply of oxygen, blood sugar, and fatty acid to the muscles,
if there is a state of peripheral circulatory insufficiency (extravasated blood
state). This leads to a shortage of energy and, as a result, calcium ions
are not accommodated in the sarcoplasmic reticula so that the muscles
remain contracted, which causes shoulder discomfort and low back pain.

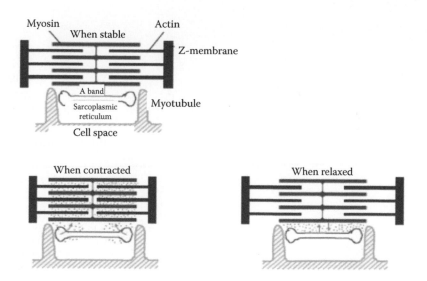

**Figure 5.3** Distribution of calcium ions in the processes of muscle contraction
and relaxation.

* *Sarcoplasmic reticulum:* A membrane-shaped structure present in muscle fibers. The endoplasmic reticula are called sarcoplasmic reticula because skeletal muscles have especially
well-developed endoplasmic reticula. An endoplasmic reticulum is an intracellular hyda-
tid or a net-like small tube that can be seen by an electron microscope.

### 5.4.4  Using glucosamine, a chitosan oligosaccharides degradation product, to improve shoulder discomfort or low back pain

The amount of blood flowing through the capillary vessels should be increased in order to improve shoulder discomfort or low back pain. The blood circulation is improved when the arterioles are expanded as the amount of blood in the capillary vessels is regulated in the arterioles (the thin arteries present before the arteries are divided into capillary vessels). The intake of chitosan oligosaccharides is expected to improve shoulder discomfort and the low back pain stemming from the muscles because glucosamine, which is a chitosan oligosaccharide degradation product, has been shown to stimulate the vagus nerves to excite the autonomic nerve center (parasympathetic nerve center) and thereby expand the arterioles.

## chapter six

# Utilization of chitin as artificial skin

## 6.1   Components and functions of the skin

In humans, the surface of the skin contains numerous hair and sweat pores, wrinkles, and different types of hair. In particular, types of hair such as downy hair are primarily round and flat, and form the stratum corneum, which is responsible for the tactile sense. The color of the skin varies depending on the amount of pigment and blood present in it. The color also depends on the fraction of light reflected from off of the skin surface or on the transparency of the skin surface. In addition to race, gender, age, and body region differences, the presence of nutritional conditions, endocrine disorders, visceral diseases, and skin diseases are important factors that have an effect on skin color.

The skin consists of the epidermis (outermost layer), dermis (inner layer), and subcutaneous tissues. Many cells constitute the skin tissue. Skin thickness varies depending on the body region in question; the thickness of the epidermis ranges from approximately 0.03 to 1.00 mm and that of the dermis is approximately 10 times more than that of the epidermis. Most of the subcutaneous tissues are formed by lipids; therefore, the thickness of the subcutaneous tissues is different at different body regions, and also varies among individuals. In the skin, many blood vessels are distributed like meshes in the dermis and subcutaneous tissues; however, there are no blood vessels in the epidermis. These blood vessels circulate blood and supply nutrients. Furthermore, the well-distributed network of sensory and autonomic nerves in the skin are responsible for the different sensations felt, the movement of smooth muscle and blood vessels, and the secretions from the sebaceous and sweat glands.

The skin is not only a characteristic of an individual but also shows the expressions of joy, anger, sorrow, and pleasure. For instance, when individuals are ashamed, their faces become pinkish; when they are angry, their faces become red; and when they are surprised, their faces become bluish. In addition, the skin feels sensations such as the sense of touch, cold, warmth, and pain according to the external stimuli applied. These feelings are transmitted from the distal end of the sensory nerves and immediately transferred for the next action.

The skin protects the body against mechanical stimuli such as beating, pressing, and friction by providing a strong and high-resistance barrier, due to the layer of thick fat tissues at the bottom and the layer of hard keratin at the top. Furthermore, the skin has fat films on its surface and is highly acidic,* thus preventing the infiltration of water and bacteria, respectively.

When it is exposed to sunlight, the skin becomes red and the concentration of pigment increases due to the ultraviolet rays of sunlight. Ultraviolet rays are harmful to the human body, and therefore, to protect the body, the skin produces melanin pigment when it absorbs ultraviolet rays. Moreover, immune bodies are also produced in the skin. Therefore, lifetime immunity is gained with the onset and resolution of rashes, such as those associated with chickenpox or smallpox; individuals who are vaccinated against such diseases are also protected.

The sweat and sebaceous glands† secrete sweat and oil, respectively, on the skin surface, making it smooth and glossy. In general, water-soluble substances are absorbed by the skin with difficulty, whereas fat- or alcohol-soluble substances are more easily assimilated. In particular, substances that are made into emulsions by adding emulsifiers can easily penetrate into the skin.

The skin is a poor conductor of warmth and blocks external high temperatures and regulates heat dissipation. Approximately 80% of the heat released from the body is generated from the skin. This action is achieved by heat conduction and dissipation and water evaporation.

As such, the skin plays various important roles such as covering the entire body, protecting important internal organs, and maintaining a constant body temperature by discharging moisture and salt.

## 6.2   Wound healing effect

When the epidermis has been destroyed due to severe lacerations, the dermis is also destroyed; therefore, the skin completely loses its ability to regenerate. Depending on the degree of damage, it may be life-threatening.

---

* *Acidity*: A measure that indicates the intensity of the acidity of solutions containing acids.
† *Sebaceous glands*: Lipid glands that are connected to the hypodermal glands and follicles of the skin, which secrete and discharge between 1 g and 2 g of sebum per day on average through the pores on the surface of the skin.

Even when the area of damage is small, if left as it is, the affected area will become colloid: specifically, a benign tumor will develop in which the skin proliferates abnormally. Above all, the ugly scars caused by burning do not disappear forever.

In such cases, auto-transplantation is the best way to heal the destroyed skin. It is a process by which skin from another region of a patient's body is transplanted to the affected area. Skin from other individuals cannot be engrafted successfully, except in the cases of enzygotic twins.

However, since the amount of transplantable skin is limited, skin regeneration with artificial skin can be a good alternative. This has become possible due to the application of chitin extracted from crab shells.

In general, wound-covering materials close to the concept of artificial skin should possess the following properties:

- Pain relief
- Prevention of drying
- Prevention of growth and proliferation of bacteria
- Prevention of loss of protein and red blood cells
- Protection of exposed tendons, blood vessels, and nerves
- Promotion of wound healing

In addition, such materials should enable simple management of wound surfaces, should be cheap, and should be mass-producible. Such wound surface-covering materials available currently include synthetic covering materials and living body covering materials, but neither of these are highly suitable for use. Synthetic covering materials cause strong foreign body reactions, have problems in bio-affinity, and can be used only for limited purposes. Living body covering materials such as the skins of pigs, sheep, and dogs have been used from old times. The living skin of pigs has been used in very limited applications, but it lacks practicality. In addition, chicken egg membranes and human amnia (a thin membrane that envelops the fetus in the uterus) can be used, but they cannot be easily bought. Currently, lyophilized pig skin and collagen are used only in some limited applications. Such defects have been sufficiently complemented while studying artificial skins made of crab shell-extracted chitin, which can be used as wound surface protectants.

## 6.3   Methods of making artificial skins

In 1970, Prudden et al. published a study suggesting the potential of chitin as a medical material. Ointments made of ground shark cartilage are involved in the early recovery of wounds; therefore, they reviewed which components of shark cartilage were contributing to the effect and found that N-acetylglucosamine played an important role. Consequently, since chitin is a constituting unit of N-acetylglucosamine, they conducted an animal experiment using chitin powder to study the relationship between chitin and wound healing.

The researchers found that as compared with in the control group, wounds that were sprayed with chitin powder healed faster. Subsequently, they molded the chitin powder into threads and films and examined their effects. However, their study was stopped before the threads and films were commercialized because the molding method was poor. Later, Unitika Central Research Laboratories of Japan investigated chitin-molded body manufacturing methods and succeeded in manufacturing high-quality products that can be used as medical materials. Much attention was focused on in this material, and animal experiments and clinical studies conducted in various fields at medical research institutes by researchers showed interesting results.

In particular, studies were concentrated on the use of chitin for wound surface protection; the use of chitin as an artificial skin in a broad sense attracted public attention, and a product named Beschitin W was developed. The manufacturing method is briefly described henceforth.

Chitin is a mucilaginous polysaccharide formed by β-1,4 binding of N-acetyl-D-glucosamine, in which only the hydroxyl group of cellulose residues has been substituted by an amino acetyl group. The calcium and protein are removed from the exoskeleton of crustaceans, such as crab and shrimp, to obtain highly pure chitin powder having ash contents <0.2%. Thereafter, the chitin powder is treated to enhance the solubility and dissolved in an acidic solvent to make a chitin solution at concentrations of approximately 10%.

While being measured, this solution is extruded through a nozzle of a micropore into an aqueous solution and then rolled on a roller at a constant speed to obtain multi-filaments with outer diameters of several microns. After sufficiently removing the residual solvent using water, the multi-filaments are cut to the lengths of approximately 5 mm, treated to increase protein adsorption, and made into initial sheets using polyvinyl alcohol as a binder (i.e., the cut filaments are made of a nonwoven fabric). The thickness measures between 100 and 120 μm. Subsequently, the sheet is sterilized using ethylene oxide gas and packed to make Beschitin W.

## 6.4 Chitin artificial skin that shows amazing effects

When transparent films were made of chitin and mouse-derived fibro-blasts (cells that are an important component of connective tissues) were proliferated on the films, accurate proliferation was shown. The state of adhesion was improved as compared with in the cellulose films, and Beschitin W was found to have no adverse effect on the proliferation of normal cells on wound surfaces, and showed good effects on the forma-tion of epidermal tissues.

Artificial skins made of chitin can be used as protectants for the major-ity of wounds. They have been used on wounds such as lacerations, donor site scars, and skin ulcers, and showed excellent outcomes in terms of analgesic effects; adhesiveness; and resistance to dissolution, drying, and the formation of the epidermis. Half-side tests (tests in which the halves of the epithelium are covered with different materials) with other similar wound covering protectants such as lyophilized pigskin, lyophilized der-mis of pigskin, collagen membranes, and bioplan (nylon fibers coated with silicone and treated with peptide) were conducted on donor sites (average length: approximately 15/1,000") at 22 university hospitals and general hospitals across the country. During the treatments, differences between the two materials studied in terms of analgesic effect, adhesion, resistance to dissolution, drying, and the formation of the epidermis were evaluated, and the amounts of leachate were compared, until the end of the treat-ments. The overall outcomes of artificial skins made of chitin were similar or better as compared with those of conventional products in 90% of the tests, indicating that the outcomes of artificial skins made of chitin were good (Figure 6.1). No side effects were observed during the treatment periods. In addition, acute toxicity, subacute toxicity, epidermis reaction, pyrogenicity, physical property, transplantation, cytotoxicity, hemolytic, mutagenicity, and antigenicity tests were conducted as safety tests, and all the tests indicated negative results and high safety (Figure 6.1).

Therefore, Beschitin W contains pre-proliferated epidermal cells as porous bodies on chitin. When it is attached to deep wounds, the com-plete epidermis is formed by the chitin, which is decomposed as epider-mis cells proliferate. Twenty years ago, Japan began to sell the artificial skin under the name Beschitin W and, at the time, was exporting it to 86 countries. If it is used more widely clinically and its characteristics are proven, it will be used not only as skin but also as a restorative material

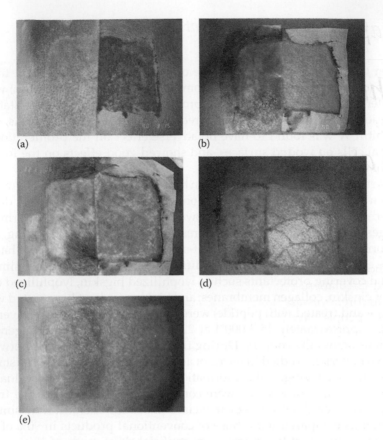

*Figure 6.1* A clinical test in which chitin artificial skin was transplanted on severely scratched wounds. Lyophilized dermis of pigskin was used as the control (a) Lyophilized dermis of pigskin (LDPS) and Beschitin W were attached to the halves of a donor site on the left femoral region of a 48-year old man, respectively, (b) Three days later, the wound surface attached with Beschitin W became a gel state so that the hemorrhage stopped well. The side attached with LDPS continued bleeding, (c) Both sides were dried by eight days later but the LDPS side has some small wet regions, (d) When the materials were taken off 12 days later, the Beschitin W became the epithelium. The LDPS side had some parts not completely cured and (e) The healing of the LDPS side was delayed and the LDPS side swelled up 20 days later. (From Kibo, H., *Medical Application of Chitin and Chitosan*, Gihoto Publishing, Tokyo, Japan, 1994.)

for damaged regions in the human body. In addition, chitin is highly likely to have its functionality enhanced by chemical modification in the future. Once this potential has been realized, chitin can also be used as a biomaterial. In the future, the chitin contained in shrimp and crab shells, which are fish processing wastes, can be used to treat skin damaged by burns or accidents without any resultant scars.

# chapter seven

# Chitosan oligosaccharides that prevent hazards due to alcohol consumption

## 7.1 Appropriate drinking is good for our health

In general, drinking moderate amounts of alcohol is good for health; however, excessive drinking is harmful. As an old representative Japanese medical book (養生訓) written in 1712 states that "drinking a little improves blood circulation, removes uncomfortable feelings, improves the stamina, and relieves anxiety, but excessive drinking harms people in many ways," people have been drinking moderately for health since old times. Even though there are many illnesses caused by overeating nowadays, an appropriate amount of alcohol can be helpful for our health (Ekiken, 1977).

In Korea, medicinal wines have been manufactured and used instead of drugs in some cases. Plum wine has an effect on diarrhea; tangerine wine is effective for fatigue recovery, arteriosclerosis; and beriberi, and *Lycium* wine supplements feebleness, removes fatigue fever (the fever that causes weakness and feebleness in the body), enhances the vital force, strengthens the waist and legs, improves the complexion, and controls tearing. Furthermore, strawberry wine is good for skin beauty and stimulates the appetite, while mulberry wine maintains youthfulness. These wines have been patronized since the old times for such efficacies.

Another option, ginseng wine, which is known to be at its best when made specifically of Korean ginseng, is effective for individuals who are in low spirits and who have low body temperatures. Korean wine is good for indigestion, and velvet antler wine is effective for individuals who easily contract the common cold because of weak bronchial tubes or lungs and those who have low stamina. Korean angelica wine is good for those who frequently feel dizzy due to severe anemia, and *Acanthopanax* wine is known to be the elixir of life together with ginseng wine and is used for neuralgia and ear reflexology. *Achyranthes* wine is made by decocting the root of *Achyranthes* grass to extract the juice and is used for troubles in the knees, other joints, or in the waist. *Rehmannia glutinosa* wine (made of a mixture of *Rehmannia glutinosa* and glutinous rice) is good for those who digest food well at normal times but who break out in a cold sweat and have dry skin or dry mouth frequently. *Poria cocos* wine (made of a mushroom that grows on pine roots underground) is effective for individuals who cannot smoothly urinate at normal times. Chrysanthemum wine is used for individuals who easily develop bloodshot eyes or who have high blood pressure, and *Polygonatum* wine (made of *Polygonatum* root) is good for recovery from all kinds of fatigue. Lastly, viper wine is widely used for neuralgia.

In general, alcohol consumption can be appropriately helpful for health and useful for the treatment of diseases. However, the appropriate amount of alcohol consumption is ambiguous and has not been quantified. Excessive consumption can lead to obesity due to the intake of excess calories. Furthermore, when alcohol is consumed excessively, it may disturb the actions of the brain, including in particular the various regulatory centers in the hypothalamus.* It may also affect blood pressure, and lead to arteriosclerosis, heart diseases, diabetes, gout, and liver diseases.

## 7.2   Effects of alcohol on the human body

The main component of various alcoholic drinks is ethyl alcohol. The unique aroma of the small amount of esters contained in alcohol gives a peculiar feeling to humans; however, their pharmacological effect is weak. The impurities of the brewing process, such as amyl alcohol and acetaldehyde, are very poisonous components and are what cause a hangover.

After drinking the same amount of alcohol, some individuals may become significantly drunk, whereas others may not become as drunk. In some Western movies, we have seen characters drinking whiskey from a bottle. In general, Caucasians are heavier drinkers than Asians. Notably, there are differences between the races that may be the cause of this. In the body, approximately 20% of the alcohol consumed is absorbed in the stomach and the remaining 80% is absorbed in the small intestine and sent to the liver. Once the alcohol has entered the stomach or the upper small intestine, it is absorbed almost entirely into the blood. From approximately five minutes after drinking alcohol, the alcohol components can be detected in the blood and, at a time of up to approximately 30 or 90 minutes later, the alcohol reaches its peak concentration in the blood and affects various physiological actions. Although alcohol is mostly metabolized in the liver and gets broken down to become water and carbonic acid gas,

---

* *Hypothalamus*: A part of the brain buried in the cerebrum that plays the most important role in controlling the internal environment of the living body in vertebrates. The hypothalamus is involved in the regulation of autonomic nerves that maintain basic body function in animals and of sexual nerves.

which are the final products, some acetaldehyde, which is an intermediate metabolite, is produced to cause a hangover. A small amount of alcohol is excreted from the body through the kidneys and lungs. The rate of alcohol metabolism is 150 mg of alcohol per kilogram of body weight per hour, which corresponds to one bottle of beer. However, the metabolism rate is slightly different among different persons. During metabolism, alcohol infiltrates into the various viscera and organs in the body and causes diverse physiological phenomena. Among the symptoms that occur after drinking, many can be attributed to the actions of acetaldehyde, while some are attributable to the actions of alcohol itself. For example, the reddening of the face or body, vomiting, and headache are attributable to the actions of acetaldehyde. Individuals who get drunk easily have a poor efficiency of acetaldehyde metabolism; therefore, acetaldehyde is accumulated in the body even when a small amount of alcohol has been consumed, leading to various unpleasant symptoms.

Although there are five types of aldehyde dehydrogenases in the liver, types I and II aldehyde dehydrogenases mainly decompose acetaldehyde. Type II aldehyde dehydrogenase is present in both Asians and Caucasians, and 50% of Asians are genetically deficient in type I aldehyde dehydrogenase, which reacts with acetaldehyde at low concentrations because of its high affinity to acetaldehyde. Therefore, many Asians get drunk easily.

## 7.2.1   Effects on the central nerves

Ethyl alcohol has a more remarkable effect on the central nervous system than any other organ in the body and acts as a repressor to the central nervous system similarly as do other anesthetics of the central nervous system. In particular, it represses the brain, which maintains and controls the functions of various organs of our body, thereby causing changes in nervous system activity in various parts of our body. Notably, it greatly affects emotional actions and mental operations.

Under the influence of alcohol, individuals express their original human desires, which are usually controlled by reason and intellect, as they feel triumphant and confident and can persuade others with diverse speech skills. However, after a while, they display immoral or unscrupulous behavior without hesitating, thereby damaging the good personality accumulated throughout their life.

In addition, they sometimes make a prompt decision on an important matter that must be seriously considered, thereby suffering a great loss. Since their senses become dull, they show poor efficiency while performing a task that requires delicate functions, or they may incur various accidents that could be avoided, thereby suffering great losses and sometimes losing precious lives.

## 7.2.2    Effects on the cardiovascular and circulatory systems

Although a small amount of alcohol may cause tachycardia (heart pulses at a rate more frequent than usual), a large amount of alcohol can cause a decline in cardiovascular functions, a decrease in myocardial contractility, and may even lead to respiratory arrest. Patients suffering from chronic alcoholism show high frequencies of myocarditis and onset of arrhythmias. When an individual is drunk, the skin color turns red and the hands and feet burn since peripheral blood vessels dilate; the drinker feels as if he/she has new power. However, the accumulated body heat radiates, gradually dropping the body temperature. Therefore, it is unreasonable to drink alcohol in winter to overcome the cold weather. In fact, such increases the possibility of frostbite and may even lead to death in some cases.

## 7.2.3    Effects on digestive organs

With respect to the digestive organs, alcohol causes disorders in gastrointestinal movements and end-exocrine functions; however, the degree of disorder depends on the concentration of alcohol consumed. Although it is said that a small amount of alcohol stimulates the secretion of saliva and gastric juice to promote appetite and help digestion, when consumed in large quantities, alcohol irritates the gastric mucosa to cause gastritis and even gastric ulcer in severe cases.

After drinking, if nausea or vomiting and severe epigastralgia occur the following morning, the individual is confirmed to have gastritis or a gastric ulcer. If the person ignores these signals of the stomach and again drinks alcohol, it is natural that the person will contract complications such as gastric ulcer and experience pain. According to experts, cases in which strong liquors directly stimulate the gastric mucosa to cause hyperemia and stomach wall inflammation, leading to the development of gastritis or gastric ulcers, can frequently be seen at clinics. Even if the appropriate amount of alcohol is consumed every time, individuals who habitually drink alcohol may suffer from constipation or diarrhea, which is a result of the loss of balance of bowel movements. If this condition continues, nutrients and vitamins are lost from the body and the health condition gradually deteriorates. Drinking is the biggest factor that causes pancreatitis. Therefore, individuals with suspected gastritis, gastric ulcer, duodenum ulcer, or pancreatitis should never drink.

## 7.2.4    Effects on the liver

The liver is an important organ that metabolizes various nutrients, detoxifies toxins, and produces blood coagulation factors. Alcohol can cause various liver diseases such as alcoholic fatty liver, alcoholic hepatitis, and alcoholic hepatic cirrhosis.

Although just vague senses of fatigue, inappetence, nausea, vomiting, and indigestion appear at the beginning, if the person ignores these symptoms and continues to drink alcohol, the diseases will gradually progress: the liver becomes swollen, jaundice develops with yellowing of the eyes and skin, and ascites are generated. In addition, the belly becomes swollen, leading to a shortage of breath; esophageal variceal hemorrhage may also occur in severe cases, leading to massive hematemesis and even bloody excrement in some instances. If the condition progresses further, the liver will become swollen and the person will develop chronic coma, which can lead to death. However, some drinkers do not want to quit drinking and take various expensive liver pills only when these symptoms have begun to appear; the possibility of recovery from such symptoms in these cases are moderate. Therefore, the importance of prevention rather than treatment should be reiterated.

### 7.2.5 Effects on the brain and renal functions

Alcohol affects both brain cells and other nervous system cells. Liver damage appeared in male drinkers ≤35 years, 19% of the drinkers had liver cirrhosis and 59% of the drinkers suffered from intellectual damage, which was evaluated using memory, concentration, and comprehension tests. Alcohol causes diuretic action because it suppresses the secretion of the antidiuretic hormone in the pituitary gland. This leads to not only a loss of water but also the loss of various electrolytes, eventually resulting in aggravated lactic acidemia,* caused by the alcohol metabolic process, and more problems.

## 7.3 Chitosan that prevents trouble due to drinking

Chitosan is involved in alcohol metabolism (Figure 7.1). Eating fatty foods during alcohol intake suppresses a rise in the alcohol concentration in the blood. Tachiyashiki and Imaizumi reported that when soybean oil was orally administered at a rate of 1 g per 1 kg of the body weight to rats 30 minutes before orally administrating alcohol at a rate of 1 g per 1 kg of the body weight, the rise in the blood alcohol concentration was suppressed. Therefore, this implies that if a certain amount of alcohol is consumed along with the intake of fatty foods, that the latter will reduce the effects of the drink in comparison with in someone who is only drinking.

---

* *Lactic acidosis*: This refers to a condition where lactic acid appears in blood because lactic acid was accumulated due to the lack of oxygen in the tissues.

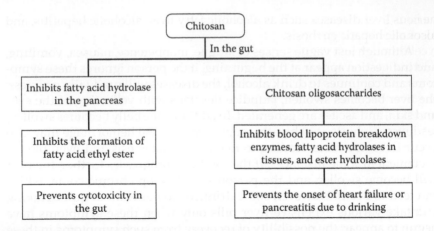

**Figure 7.1** Chitin, chitosan, and alcohol.

However, the reason why such a phenomenon occurs had not been clearly identified until recently. Dr. Tsujita's et al. (2004) study helped provide an explanation of this phenomenon. In the process of studying fatty acid-degrading enzymes, he found that hydrolysis occurs when water is present. However, the involved enzymes degrade fat, and the fatty acid generated by the degradation becomes alcohol, producing fatty acid ethyl ester when alcohol is present, instead of water. As shown in Figure 7.1, when the fat in a meal is degraded by a fatty acid-degrading enzyme secreted from the pancreas, an acyl-enzyme complex is formed as an intermediate product.

In this case, if water is present, the complex will be hydrolyzed to produce fatty acid. This is a known as the hydrolysis reaction. Some of the fatty acid produced is absorbed by the epithelial cells.

However, what happens if fatty foods are eaten while alcohol is drunk? Since fat and water are incompatible with each other, they do not mix with each other. Fat has a higher affinity to alcohol than to water. Therefore, ethanol is gathered around the fat. When the fatty acid-degrading enzyme acts on the fat and ethanol, the fatty acid in the acyl-enzyme complex is transferred to ethanol to produce a fatty acid ethyl ester. This phenomenon is called alcohol-added degradation.

The fatty acid ethyl ester produced is not absorbed into the epithelial cells; they are instead mostly excreted into the stomach. Eventually, since alcohol is combined with fatty acid and excreted in feces, the blood alcohol concentration does not rise very much and the drinker becomes less drunk. Fatty acid ethyl ester synthesis occurs not only in the gut but also in the blood and tissues. Fatty acid ethyl ester is also synthesized by lipoprotein degradation enzymes involved in the blood lipoprotein metabolism and is produced by fatty acid-degrading enzymes and ester hydrolases in the heart or pancreas, which have less alcohol dehydrogenase that decomposes alcohol. However, fatty acid ester inhibits mitochondrial respiration in cells and causes cell destruction, resulting in heart failure (a state of circulatory failure that presents various clinical symptoms) or pancreatitis. To prevent alcohol from being absorbed in the intestines, alcohol should be converted to fatty acid ethyl ester; however, the fatty acid ester produced in the cells is toxic.

## 7.4   Chitosan that makes people get drunk quickly

Although chitosan inhibits the reactions of fatty acid hydrolase in the pancreas and hinders the absorption of fat in the intestines, there is a possibility of it also affecting the synthesis of fatty acid ethyl esters. In some cases, the intake of chitosan when drinking alcohol along with eating fatty snacks may in fact induce the drinker to get drunk faster. Although there are diverse opinions on whether this phenomenon is good for the body, given that this phenomenon inhibits the production of fatty acid ethyl ester, which is likely to do harm to the cells in the gut, it can be regarded to be a desirable phenomenon.

Since chitosan oligosaccharides can be absorbed into the body and inhibit the production of fatty acid ethyl esters in the heart or pancreas after drinking to prevent heart failure or pancreatitis, the intake of chitosan oligosaccharides during drinking may prevent drinking-induced hazards.

# chapter eight

# Chitosan oligosaccharides in dentistry and systemic diseases

The teeth are important structures that represent the first line of the food digestion and absorption process. This process starts in the mouth when food is chewed by the teeth. When teeth are damaged, it is difficult to chew food, causing gastrointestinal disorders. Even if only one of the 32 teeth is lost, there is a change in the pressure applied to each tooth, damaging the health of the entire mouth and leading to abnormalities such as those of the gums and jawbones. With the increasing standard of living, the interest in health has also been growing among many people. However, dental health remains neglected in most cases. In the last two decades, the incidence of tooth decay in South Korean children has increased by at least four times due to the spread of fast food, carbonic acid drinks, and soft and light food-centered dietary habits. After eating food, carbohydrate debris often gets stuck in the gaps between the teeth. Oral bacteria act on these carbohydrates, leading to decay (fermentation) and acid production. This acid dissolves the mineral component on the surfaces of the teeth, leading to dental caries. The continuous growth of oral bacteria on tooth surfaces leads to plaque formation and inflammation around the gums. In general, 1 g of plaque contains approximately 200 million bacteria, and it is a major cause of gingivitis, periodontitis, and cavities. In particular, plaque in regions inaccessible with a toothbrush becomes hard and forms dental plaque over time. Oral diseases can be prevented by blocking only one of the following steps:

Food intake → Plaque formation → Dental plaque formation

## 8.1 Harmful bacteria in the mouth

The human mouth offers a good environment for bacterial reproduction because of the presence of adequate moisture, nutrients, and suitable temperatures. Therefore, a group of microorganisms called oral residents live in the human mouth. These oral residents are comprised of >700 species of microorganisms including many unidentified bacteria that are comparable to intestinal bacteria. The primary habitat for these microbes is the dental plaque formed in the gums; the density of bacteria here is much higher than that in feces. Every 1 mL of saliva contains approximately $10^{8-9}$ bacteria and every 1 g of mature plaque contains approximately $10^{10-11}$ bacteria.

However, strong pathogenic bacteria are not detected in oral microbiota. In cases in which oral hygiene is well-managed, the microbiota strives to maintain the oral environment and a good symbiotic relationship with the host. In general, bacterial invasions in the oral mucosa cause mild inflammations; however, the oral mucosa is more resistant to bacterial invasion or inflammation than the intestinal mucosa in many ways. Moreover, an increase in the amount of plaque due to a lack of oral hygiene results in the growth of periodontal pathogens that lead to metastasis to a pathogenic plaque. Therefore, chronic inflammatory diseases may occur that lead to organic and functional disorders of the living body. In addition, there is a decline in the defense mechanism, leading to periodontal diseases.

*Streptococcus* spp. are most frequently detected in all parts of the oral cavity and are the major cause of dental caries, as they aid in the formation of dental plaque through the production of glucan. In the field of dentistry and medicine, *Streptococcus* spp. have attracted much attention because they cause infectious diseases such as dental caries, periodontal diseases, infectious endocarditis, and pneumonia. Some of these bacteria are harmless to the human body, but those that reproduce in the plaque attached to the tooth surface are harmful. In addition, the spread of harmful bacteria through the blood may cause endocarditis, arthritis, rheumatism, pneumonia, heart disease, and paranasal sinusitis.

Dental erosion, often known as dental caries, is a disease that occurs in the hard tissues of teeth. Dental erosion occurs because the teeth surfaces are corroded, and the minerals are leached by the acid generated by the corrosive bacteria in the oral cavity. The causative bacteria *Streptococcus mutans* that cause dental caries produce dextran, leading to the formation of membrane-like structures on the tooth surface. Since dextran is very sticky, other bacteria or food debris easily sticks to it to form plaque, which is a cluster of bacteria.

The bacteria in this plaque produce acids from the sugars present in food; these acids infiltrate into the surfaces of the teeth, dissolve the enamel, and destroy the dentin beneath it. Periodontal disease is a condition where food debris, plaque, and dental plaque (which is hardened and calcified plaque) are jammed in small pockets called periodontal pockets between the teeth and surrounding tissues, causing inflammations.

The onset of gum diseases is also common after the common cold. The number of patients who visit hospitals due to gum diseases has been increasing by >20% every year. According to the Health Insurance Review and Assessment Service, 12,896,270 patients with gum disease visited hospitals in 2014. Gum diseases occur when oral bacteria eat the food debris in the spaces between the teeth and gums and reproduce. Due to bacterial reproduction, white blood cells gather in that area, causing inflammation. In severe inflammation, the bacteria penetrate into the blood vessels by attacking the gum bones and thereby assaulting the entire body.

Therefore, the presence of gum diseases can increase the risk of vascular diseases. Studies on gum diseases have shown that the presence of a gum disease increases the risk of occurrence of coronary artery diseases by 14% and that of cerebral infarction by 111%. In pregnant women with a gum disease, inflammation-generated toxins affect the secretion of the hormone necessary for the contraction of the uterus, leading to premature birth.

In addition, the presence of gum diseases facilitates the onset of diabetes, resulting in further complications. A research team from the College of Medicine, Columbia University, United States, followed 9,296 general people without diabetes at the start of the study period for 17 years and found that diabetes occurred two-folds more frequently in the individuals who had periodontal diseases (Soskolne and Klinger, 2001). The bacterium, *Gingivalis*, that causes gum diseases passes into the blood vessels and results in inflammation and hindering of vascular functions; this leads to glucose metabolic abnormalities.

Diabetes patients with gum diseases have between four and six times higher risks of diabetes complications and poor blood sugar control, respectively, because their wounds do not easily heal and their recovery from injuries is slow. Due to the gum disease, food is not chewed properly; thus, it is poorly digested in the body and the nutrients contained within it are not well-absorbed, making it difficult for blood sugar to be controlled. When their blood sugar is not properly managed, an individual again becomes susceptible to gum diseases; this vicious circle is continuous. Since gum diseases are lifestyle diseases that occur when the teeth are not properly managed, having good lifestyle habits is of paramount importance. To prevent gum diseases, the places where bacteria can easily grow, such as the gingival sulcus, should be intensively eliminated and the food residues stuck between the teeth should be removed using an interdental toothbrush or dental floss. The plaque becomes dental plaque when it is hardened, and dental plaque should be removed by scaling.

Bad breath or bad smell from the mouth can cause displeasure to the surrounding people, leading to encumbrances in social life. Bad breath can be caused by oral health problems, by an impairment in other organs, or have a number of other systemic causes. Oral health problems include poor management of prosthetic appliances in the mouth, poor management of the oral environment, and the onset of diseases such as dental erosion, periodontal disease, stomatitis, and oral cancer. Systemic diseases include rhinitis, gastritis, bronchitis, liver diseases, and diabetes. In general, bad breath can be prevented by cleansing the oral environment (specifically by brushing the teeth and cleaning the tongue after eating and before going to bed).

## 8.2   Oral infection and systemic diseases

Sakamoto (2010) explains that in the 1970s, bacterial translocation, in the field of medicine, was defined as "the transfer of living bacteria from the alimentary canal to the lymph nodes,* liver, spleen, or other organs." Later, the definition was updated to include pathological conditions due to endotoxin and exotoxin translocations and toxin-stimulated cytokines (physiological active proteins released from blood cells).

Since old times, the concept of *dental focal infection* has been known of in the dental field because secondary diseases are caused in distant organs by periodontal diseases such as gingivitis in chronic regional lesions (regional chronic inflammations with bacteria), chronic periodontitis, pulpitis (inflammations occurring in teeth) caused by dental caries, and proximal periodontitis. For example, infectious heart endocarditis is caused by oral bacteria, which settle down in the endocardium.

Oral bacteria can cause secondary diseases by the following three mechanisms:

- Infections due to mouth-derived bacterial dislocation that induces bacteremia, including bacterial endocarditis, acute bacterial myocarditis, brain tumor, cavernous thrombosis of the sinus, paranasal sinusitis, lung abscess/lung infection, skin ulcer, osteomyelitis, and artificial joint infection
- Metastatic disorders due to toxin circulation by oral bacteria, including cerebral infarction, acute myocardial infarction, abnormal delivery (low-birth-weight infant delivery), persistent fever, sudden tertiary neuralgia, addictive shock syndrome, systemic granulocyte defects, and chronic periostitis
- Metastatic inflammation due to an impaired immune function stemming from oral bacteria, including Behcet's disease,[†] chronic urticaria, inflammatory bowel disease, Crohn's disease, and proliferative brain disease

## 8.3   Effects of mouth care on influenza virus infection

Sialylated hydrolase (neuraminidase [NA]) produced by oral bacteria can reduce the effect of anti-influenza drugs by promoting influenza virus infection. Professional mouth care is emerging as an effective

---

* *Lymph node*: An organ in the mammalian lymphatic system that captures foreign substances in tissues and lymph to conduct immune responses.
† *Behcet's disease*: A disease wherein the major symptoms are recurrent aphthous ulcer and iritis in the oral mucosa and the vulva.

countermeasure against influenza. The increasing prevalence of influenza that presents every year has become a great threat in South Korea, which has become a super-aged society. Influenza aggravates into a severe disease in individuals who have any other underlying disease. It is essential to prepare for the emergence of new viruses because global pandemic diseases caused by new influenza viruses may cause serious health-related damage and lead to social disorder.

The morbidity and mortality rates in individuals with Spanish influenza who also had an oral disease were two to four times higher than those in those with no disease. In addition, periodontal pathogenic bacteria that exist in the mouth were detected in the lungs of individuals infected with influenza (A/H1N1 pdm09), which prevailed largely in 2009. Furthermore, oral bacteria promote the release of viruses, spreading infection with influenza viruses.

Oral care is very effective in preventing pneumonia caused by oral bacteria; the importance of oral care has been recognized in clinics because regular oral care can reduce postoperative infection, thereby enabling early discharge of patients.

Bacteria (such as *Streptococcus mitis* and *Streptococcus oralis*) that promote influenza virus infection are the most prevalent bacterial species in dental plaque and are detected in the throat and airway at very high frequencies. An epidemiological survey was conducted by Abe et al. (2006) to study the effects of oral care on the onset of influenza by dividing elderly persons into two groups: group 1 received professional oral care from dental hygienists once per week, while group 2 did not receive any care. They reviewed the relationship between the NA and trypsin-like protease (TLP) activities in the saliva and the onset rates of influenza. NA and TLP activities in the saliva decreased in the group that received professional oral care as compared with in the group that did not receive any care. During the intervention period, one out of 98 subjects (1.0%) in the group that received professional oral care was diagnosed with influenza, whereas nine out of 92 subjects (9.8%) in the group that did not receive any care were diagnosed with influenza. In conclusion, professional oral care inhibited the NA and TLP activities in the saliva, making the oral environment nonconducive for viral infections, thereby preventing the onset of influenza.

NA-generated oral bacteria promote influenza virus infection and significantly reduce the effect of anti-influenza drugs. Therefore, maintaining a clean oral environment with professional mouth care is effective for the prevention of influenza and pneumonia. In addition, mouth care does not require a large amount of research funding as is often required for vaccine development. Furthermore, it does not have a risk of side effects and can adequately be used as a countermeasure against new viruses because it can easily prevent influenza nonspecifically to antigens.

***Table 8.1*** Representative oral bacteria

| Bacteria in the normal oral cavity | Periodontal pathogenic bacteria | Dental caries-causing bacteria |
| --- | --- | --- |
| *Streptococcus mitis* | *Porphyromonas gingivalis* | *Streptococcus mutans* |
| *Streptococcus thermophilus* | *Tannerella forsythia* | *Streptococcus sobrinus* |
| *Actinomyces israelii* | *Treponema denticola* | *Lactobacillus* |
| *Actinomyces meyeri* | *Aggregatibacter actinomycetemcomitans* | |
| | *Fusobacterium nucleatum* | |

## 8.4　Oral microorganisms and cancer

Many reports have indicated that numerous residents or viruses are present in the oral cavity and that they cause various diseases.

Multiple bacteria exist in the mouth that comprise the bacterial flora present (Table 8.1). *Streptococcus* and *Actinomyces* are the predominant bacteria in the normal state. An increase in the periodontal pathogenic bacteria results in periodontal disease, which is one of the two major diseases of the oral cavity. In periodontal disease, the gingival junctional epithelium proliferates and moves in the direction of myodiastasis, deepening the periodontal pockets and possibly destroying the periodontal tissues. This can lead to a loss of the teeth. According to epidemiological surveys (Miyazaki et al., 2015), patients with periodontal disease often have high carcinogenesis rates, regardless of whether or not they smoke or drink; these studies also suggest that periodontal disease is an independent risk factor for cancer. In addition, periodontal pathogenic bacteria, human papilloma virus,[*] and *Epstein-Barr* virus[†] are some of the causes of carcinogenesis and cancer progression.

## 8.5　Periodontal disease and diabetes

Periodontal disease occurs more frequently, and demonstrates a faster disease progression, in diabetic patients. Furthermore, the risk of its recurrence is higher in diabetic patients than in non-diabetic patients. Therefore, it is also known as the sixth complication of diabetes. This

---

[*] *Human papilloma virus*: A deoxyribonucleic acid (DNA) virus that causes papillomas in humans, cows, dogs, and rabbits.

[†] *Epstein-Barr virus*: A DNA virus belonging to the gamma herpes virus subfamily in the herpes family. It is a pathogenic agent of infectious mononucleosis, and it is suspected to be related with Burt's lymphoma and epipharyngeal carcinoma. It causes infinite proliferative transformation of human B lymphocytes.

can be attributed to the fact that inflammations occur more severely in diabetic patients as compared with in non-diabetic patients. High blood sugar or obesity due to diabetes leads to the progression of periodontal tissue destruction, which in turn aggravates periodontal inflammations. Recently, it has been estimated that in Japan, approximately 20% of diabetic patients with periodontal disease are suffering from systemic inflammations that make the periodontal disease more problematic. Since inflammations due to periodontal disease eventually spread throughout the entire body, the progression of inflammations should be suppressed before they become severe. Hence, maintaining blood sugar control is important to avoid other complications. In general, if glycated hemoglobin (HbA1c) is maintained below 7%, the progression of periodontal disease will be inhibited, similarly as in the case of non-diabetic patients. It is also important to maintain HbA1c <7% to reduce the risk of recurrence of periodontal disease. Obesity and smoking also affect the onset and progression of periodontal disease. Therefore, general risk factors for lifestyle diseases should be managed. However, in cases where periodontal disease has become severe because the progression of periodontal disease could not be easily inhibited, it causes mild inflammations in the body and affects diabetes.

Periodontal disease is significantly more severe in patients with type 1 and type 2 diabetes. Approximately 10% of young patients with type 1 diabetes were found to have periodontitis, whereas only 1% of healthy persons in the same age group had periodontitis. In addition, many studies have indicated that the frequency of occurrence of periodontal disease is higher among patients with type 2 diabetes than among those with no diabetes.

A study by Nelson et al. (1990) on blood sugar control status and periodontal disease severity conducted in the United States showed that the odds ratio of periodontal disease severity (a concept of comparative risk representing, in this case, an estimate of periodontal disease incidence) was 2.90 among patients with type 2 diabetes and HbA1c ≥9.0% and 1.56 among those with HbA1c <9.0%.

Many studies have reported that periodontal disease affects the onset and management of diabetes. A study of immunity conducted in Japan (Yamagishi, 2017) reported that the prevalence of periodontal disease was significantly higher among patients who were detected as having abnormal glucose tolerance test results in the last 10 years than in those who were not detected as having abnormal glucose tolerance test results. According to a survey conducted in the United States, the prevalence of diabetes among patients with periodontal disease was approximately two times higher than that in those without periodontal disease. As such, the presence of periodontal disease increases various diabetes complications, total fat mass, and incidences of kidney and ischemic heart diseases.

## 8.6    Gum disease prevention by chitosan oligosaccharides

Gum disease is an inflammatory disease that is primarily caused by oral bacteria. Therefore, removing the causative bacteria is the most important prevention method. Approximately 58% of the bacteria can be removed by brushing. However, the complete elimination of bacteria cannot be achieved only by brushing, and this is an issue. In Japan, it has been suggested that dental caries among children could substantially be decreased if children in elementary schools were encouraged to regularly drink green tea after eating lunch. This is because green tea contains antimicrobial agents.

In a study by Park et al. (2004), the antimicrobial effects of chitosan and its oligosaccharides were tested against various bacteria. Chitosan and macromolecule oligosaccharides showed 100% antimicrobial effects against *S. mutans* that causes dental caries, whereas it showed at least 99% antimicrobial effects against low-molecular oligosaccharides. In addition, the minimal inhibitory concentration for bacterial growth was 0.06%, indicating that chitosan and its oligosaccharides can kill dental caries-causing bacteria, even at low concentrations. Therefore, rinsing with and drinking chitosan oligosaccharides solutions after eating will aid in the prevention of dental caries (Table 8.2, Figure 8.1).

Professor Hayashi from Nagasaki University examined the effects of mouthwashes and gums containing chitosan oligosaccharides on oral bacteria and found that when mouthwash was used, the total number of bacteria slightly decreased. However, the number of dental caries-causing bacteria (*S. mutans*) decreased substantially. Dental caries-causing bacteria decreased significantly more when using gums containing 2% chitosan

*Table 8.2* The antimicrobial activity of chitosan oligosaccharides against bacteria

| Gram-positive (+) bacteria | Antimicrobial activity (%) | | | |
|---|---|---|---|---|
| | Chitosan | COS I (macromolecule) | COS II (mesomolecule) | COS III (small molecule) |
| *Streptococcus mutans* | 100 | 100 | 99 | 99 |
| *Micrococcus luteus* | >99 | 70 | 67 | 63 |
| *Staphylococcus aureus* | 100 | 97 | 95 | 93 |
| *Staphylococcus epidermidis* | >99 | 82 | 57 | 23 |
| *Bacillus subtilis* | 98 | 63 | 60 | 63 |

COS: chitosan oligosaccharides.

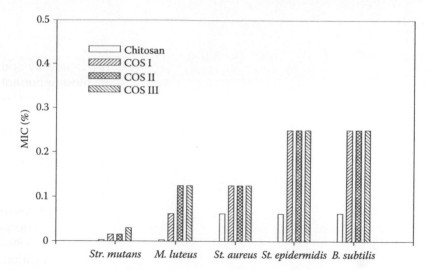

***Figure 8.1*** Minimal inhibitory concentrations of chitosan oligosaccharides against dental caries causing bacteria (*S. mutans*); COS I: 5–10 kDa; COS II: 1–5 kDa; COS III: <1 kDa.

oligosaccharides than that when using a mouthwash, indicating that the gums can prevent dental caries (Figure 8.2).

In addition, Professor Hayashi reported that when 2.5 g gums containing xylitol were compared with gums containing 2% chitosan, dental caries-causing bacteria were more significantly reduced when using the latter.

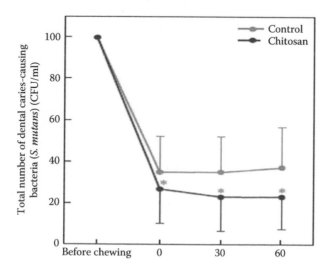

***Figure 8.2*** The reducing effect of gums containing chitosan on dental caries-causing bacteria.

## chapter nine

# Alzheimer dementia and chitosan oligosaccharides

The term *dementia* is derived from Latin and implies a *frantic state of mind*. Unlike *mental retardation*, which denotes abnormal brain functions that are present from the time of birth, dementia refers to a disease caused by damage to brain functions due to different causes, in which the patient's cognitive ability slowly declines, eventually causing difficulties in the normal life. Dementia is divided according to the possible causes into several diseases into Alzheimer's disease, which results from brain damage caused by deformation of substances in the brain; cerebrovascular infarction; vascular dementia due to hemorrhage; and degenerative brain diseases such as Parkinson's disease. Alzheimer's disease accounts for approximately 50% of cases of dementia, followed by vascular dementia (30%) due to cerebrovascular disease, degenerative brain diseases other than Alzheimer's disease (10%), and other causes (10%).

Dementia is a term that comprehensively refers to conditions in which the brain has been damaged due to diverse causes, leading to declines in functions in various areas such as memory, language ability, judgment ability, and time- and space-grasping ability, disturbing the individual's daily life. The presence of dementia can be judged only by a specialist in the absence of any special examination. However, neuropsychological tests can be used to ascertain the types of degraded cognitive functions, their severity, and the stage of advancement.

Dementia can be caused by approximately 70 diverse brain and internal diseases. Among them, the most common cause is Alzheimer's disease, which can be diagnosed through brain magnetic resonance imaging (MRI). Paradoxically, the presence of Alzheimer's disease does not yield a clear abnormality in the brain MRI. The diagnosis of Alzheimer's disease is primarily made when symptoms indicative of Alzheimer's disease are present, and other brain diseases such as cerebral infarction, brain hemorrhage, brain damage, and brain tumor are not visible in the brain MRI.

Alzheimer's disease is the most common disease that causes dementia in elderly populations. Alzheimer's disease, which usually occurs at ages >65 years and occasionally at ages between the forties and fifties, is named after German psychiatrist and neuropathologist Alois Alzheimer. Shortly after the start of the twentieth century, he observed the brain tissues of a woman who died of a cranial nerve disease, which was very rare at that time. While examining the brain tissues, he discovered that some abnormal substances had agglomerated and clustered in the tissues and that the nerve fibers had become entangled in the neurons.

The symptoms of Alzheimer's disease progress slowly initially and then gradually advance faster. Initially, the memory of recent matters primarily decreases and abnormalities in other cognitive functions such as language function and judgment accompany the symptom. In addition, in the process of the progression of the symptoms, systemic behavioral symptoms such as confusion, doubt, depression, fear or anxiety, increased aggression, and sleep disorder are involved. At the terminal stage, signs of neuropathy, such as stiffening and gait abnormalities, and physical complications, such as bedsores and infection, appear.

South Korea has been considered an aging society since the 2000s and is expected to become an aged society, where the ratio of people aged ≥65 years exceeds 14%, by 2018, and a super-aged society, where the ratio of people aged ≥65 years exceeds 20%, by 2026. At this point, dementia can be said to be the most problematic example among the senile diseases in terms of both affecting individuals and society as a whole.

The global prevalence of Alzheimer's disease among elderly persons aged ≥65 years is known to be approximately ≥5%, and this prevalence increases approximately two-fold every time the age increases by 5 years beginning at 65 years of age to become as high as 30% to 50% among elderly persons aged at least 85 years. Therefore, the number of patients and their family members suffering from dementia is expected to increase.

According to the 2012 National Dementia Epidemiology Survey announced by the Ministry of Health and Welfare, in a 2014 press release, the number of dementia patients in South Korea has been growing. The number of dementia patients, which was 470,000 in 2010, increased by 70,000 in two years to 540,000 in 2012. It is estimated that the number of dementia patients would reach 1.27 million in 2030 and 2.71 million in 2050. In 2012, in South Korea, the ratio of dementia patients with Alzheimer's disease and those with vascular dementia was 71.3% and 16.9%, respectively. According to the 2013 Annual Report presented by the Central Dementia Center, in South Korea, one out of every 10 people aged 65 to 69 years have dementia and three to four of every 10 people aged ≥85 years have dementia (Medical Observer, 2015). Dementia has become a serious problem in South Korean society only recently. The rapid increase in the elderly population along with low fertility rates indicates that the number of dementia patients that must be supported by future generations will increase in the future, which means that facilities and institutions for dementia patients should be well-equipped.

Dementia is not just a problem of the patient. Family members must also give up normal social and economic activities to care for a dementia patient, who changes over time to become like a child. In addition, the annual medical expenses per patient with dementia is $2,600, which is larger than those of hypertension ($430), cardiovascular disease ($1,320), and cerebrovascular disease ($2,050). Many dementia patients, especially those in later stages of the disease, cannot bear such substantial economic burdens on their own.

## 9.1    Alzheimer's dementia onset mechanism

As Dr. Alzheimer observed, Alzheimer's dementia is characterized by the accumulation of the plaque of a protein called β-amyloid[*] and the formation of nerve fiber tangles of TAU protein.[†] Before evaluating the question *how do these phenomena happen?*, let's briefly consider the structure of the brain (Figure 9.1).

In the human brain, a vast number of nerve cells (neurons) constitute nerves that form spider web-like networks. A neuron consist of a soma that contains a nucleus, dendrites[‡] that extend like twigs around the soma to receive signals sent by multiple adjacent neurons, and axons (nerve cells' protrusions that transfer nerve impulses from the soma to other nerve

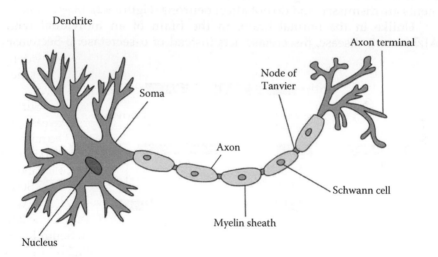

*Figure 9.1* The structure of a neuron—a typical nerve cell existing in the brain. (From https://en.wikipedia.org/wiki/File:Neuron_Hand-tuned.svg.)

---

[*] *Amyloid*: A type of glycoprotein that is formed in areas such as the brain, kidneys, and pancreas, due to chronic febrile diseases.

[†] *Tau protein*: A type of microtubule-associated protein composed of several isoforms of 50 to 60 kDa. It is abundant in the central nervous system, especially in the axon, and is also distributed in the nerve cell bodies and dendrites.

[‡] *Dendrite*: A short fiber extending from a cell body that receives information from other neurons, which it transfers to the cell body.

cells), which are necessary for the transmission of the electrical signals received from one neuron to another. The neurons exchange information with each other through electrical signals. In this case, a neuron's axon terminal and another neuron's dendrite are connected to make a synapse.

In fact, the aforementioned axon terminal and dendrite can be regarded as located adjacent to one another, rather than being connected to each other. The axon terminal and dendrite are very slightly situated away from each other at the synaptic part, where electrical signals are converted into neurotransmitters* and transmitted from the axon terminal to the dendrite (the neuron explained here is not an electric neuron but rather a chemical neuron). Although this signaling process is implemented smoothly in a healthy brain, it is impaired in the brain of a patient with Alzheimer's disease due to external and internal changes in the nerve cells.

In neurons, α-secretase and γ-secretase act together to remove the amyloid precursor protein (APP) penetrating the double lipid layers of neuron membranes. α-Secretase cleaves a part of the APP, inhibiting the formation of the β-amyloid protein. This cleaved part is liberated from the neuronal surface and the remaining part of the APP is cut by γ-secretase and discharged to the outside of the neuron. These APP fragments are dismissed and do not affect neurons (Figure 9.2).

Unlike in the normal brain, in the brain of an individual with Alzheimer's disease, β-secretase acts instead of α-secretase. β-Secretase

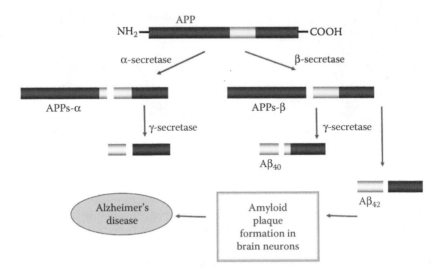

*Figure 9.2* The removal of APP in the normal brain (left) and in the brain of a patient with Alzheimer's disease (right).

* *Neurotransmitter:* A substance involved in information transmission in the nervous system, which is biosynthesized by nerve cells, stored at the axon terminal, and released when excited.

also cleaves the APP, but does so at a different part. Immediately after that, γ-secretase cleaves the remaining APP, releasing the β-amyloid protein outside of the cell membrane. β-amyloid molecules accumulate together to form oligomers outside the neuron and block the synapse, which is the site through which signals are transmitted between neurons. Hence, it not only inhibits the signal transmission but also activates immune cells and triggers an inflammatory response against dying cells. These oligomers* gather to form a β-amyloid plaque, which is comprised of accumulated amyloid protein and its oligomers.

Small tubes known as microtubules exist inside the dendrites and axons, which function as structural supports, and are responsible for the transmission of neurotransmitters (neurotransmitter vesicles). The form of these microtubules is maintained by *Tau proteins*, which play the role of an adhesive. However, in the brain neurons of Alzheimer patients, Tau proteins are detached from the microtubules, leading to their degradation. In addition, the released Tau protein molecules agglomerate together through the hyperphosphorylation process to form nerve fibers, which again agglomerate together to form neurofibrillary tangles. Consequently, the axons and dendrites of the neurons are reduced, resulting in a disconnection between adjacent nerve cells and the signals not being properly transmitted.

## 9.2   Prevention of Alzheimer's disease by chitosan oligosaccharides

Oligosaccharides (hereinafter, chito-oligosaccharides) were produced by removing the acetyl functional groups from chitin, which is a polysaccharide that exists in crustaceans such as crabs and shrimps. In addition, experiments were conducted to prove that chito-oligosaccharides inhibit the activity of β-secretase, which is an enzyme involved in the production of β-amyloid, which is a dementia-inducing substance.

Interestingly, the degree of β-secretase inhibition was dependent on the degree of deacetylation (the degree to which acetyl groups were detached from chitin). The inhibitory effect of chito-oligosaccharides was much higher when the degree of deacetylation was 90% as compared with when it was 50% or 70% (Figure 9.3). In addition, the degree of inhibition of β-secretase by 90% deacetylated chito-oligosaccharides of different molecular weights was measured. According to the results, the degree of inhibition of 90% deacetylated chito-oligosaccharides with molecular weights of 3 to 5 kDa was outstanding (Figure 9.4).

---

* *Oligomer*: Polymers with small numbers of monomers, which are basic constituents of polymers, such as oligosaccharides, oligopeptides, and oligonucleotides.

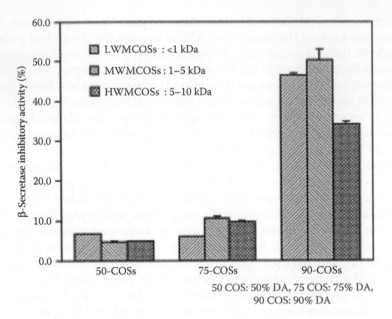

*Figure 9.3* The inhibitory effects of β-secretase according to the degree of chito-oligosaccharide deacetylation.

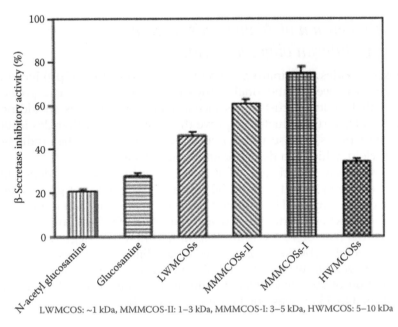

*Figure 9.4* The inhibitory effects on β-secretase of 90% deacetylated chito-oligosaccharides of different molecular weights.

However, since the degree of deacetylation of chitosan and the molecular weight of oligosaccharides are closely related with various physiological activities, they should be taken into consideration during the production of chito-oligosaccharides.

## chapter ten

# Obesity and fisheries products

According to the National Bureau of Economic Research estimates, the economic losses due to obesity cost up to $2 trillion annually (Dobbs et al., 2014). Furthermore, the magnitude of the obese and overweight population is as large as 2.1 billion individuals (30% of the world population); therefore, the sum of money spent on obesity and related issues is equivalent to the annual gross domestic product of a country such as India.

According to the Organization for Economic Cooperation and Development survey conducted in 2012, nearly half of the world's population may suffer from the problem of overweightedness by 2020 (Obesity Update 2012). In the United States, about 65% of the total population is already overweight and this ratio is expected to go up to 75% by 2020. Currently, almost 30% of the population in South Korea is overweight, but this figure may rise to 35% by 2020 and, eventually, it will be similar to the present ratios in France, Italy, and Australia. This indicates that South Korea is also not safe from obesity and other related problems, such as diabetes. In a similar vein, Asians such as South Koreans are more vulnerable to developing diabetes because the amount of insulin-producing β cells, which are essential for calorie consumption, is nearly 50% less in Asians than in Americans or Europeans. Some researchers correlate this with the consumption of rice as a staple food; however, the actual reason is yet to be ascertained.

Since obesity has emerged as one of the most serious threats to the global economy, there have been various remarkable reports published. Notably, this problem was not only observed in the United States but also in Sweden, where equality and welfare are regarded as very important; Obesity Update 2012 also indicated that fat individuals there are disadvantaged in remunerations, and so on.

There are instances that arose in which young people could not properly express confidence or a challenging spirit due to their overweightedness or obesity and were deprived of promotions. The Australian government classifies obesity as a major factor that lowers people's quality of life.

Obesity refers to a condition where more than the average amount of fat gets accumulated in the fat cells (lipocytes or adipocytes) in the fatty tissues. The surfaces of the fat masses in the fat cells exist in the form of oil droplets covered with phospholipids or proteins such as lecithin. The fat content is not constant, as there is generally a continuous synthesis and/or partial degradation; however, the imbalance between these two leads to abnormal fat accumulation in certain cases.

Obesity refers to a state in which more than the essential amount of fat has been accumulated in the body with the body mass index (BMI) exceeding 25. Overweight, on the other hand, refers to cases in which the BMI is between 23 and 24. However, a high BMI is not problematic as long as the volume of muscles in the body is largely due to physical exercises. Therefore, the professionals suggest that the degree of obesity should be determined based on the proportion of fat in relation with the total body composition test rather than just on the individual's BMI.

## 10.1   Lipogenesis in fat cells

There are two pathways for the synthesis of fats: the glucose pathway and the lipoprotein pathway. Lipoprotein* is divided into four types: chylomicron[†] (lipoprotein synthesized by the binding of long-chain fatty acids absorbed in the small intestine to proteins in the cells of the small intestine); very low-density lipoprotein (VLDL); low-density lipoprotein; and high-density lipoprotein. In the case of lipoprotein, the fat content decreases and the specific gravity increases as the protein content increases.

In the glucose pathway, the glucose (blood sugar) in the blood enters the lipocytes with the help of insulin and undergoes glycolysis to form α-glycerophosphate and pyruvate. This pyruvate forms citric acid in mitochondria and is transferred back to the cytoplasm, where the following changes occur: citric acid → acetyl coenzyme A (CoA) → acyl CoA. The acetyl CoA is bound to β-glycerophosphate to form fat (lipid) (Figure 10.1).

In the lipoprotein pathway, the lipoprotein (chylomicron, VLDL) that contains a large amount of fat is degraded into fatty acid and glycerol by the action of the lipoprotein fatty acid hydrolase (lipase) present in the wall of blood vessels. The glycerol is mainly metabolized in the liver and the fatty acid that has about 90% of the energy (kcal/g) is transported out of the blood vessels to the fat cells to form acyl CoA, which combines with glucose-derived β-glycerophosphate and synthesizes fat.

The fat is synthesized in the lipocytes in the form of oil drops, and the fat remains present in the center, whereas the phospholipids such as lecithin is present on the surface. It is structurally similar to lipoprotein. Although the lipase enzyme is present in the cytoplasm around the oil drop, lipolysis does not occur due to the presence of a lecithin monolayer on the surface, which prevents the lipase from binding with the oil drop's

---

* *Lipoprotein*: A complex of lipids and proteins represented by cholesterol, phospholipids, triglycerides, and free fatty acids.
† *Chylomicron*: Colloidal lipid granules in the blood and lymphatic fluid that act for fat transport in the small intestine. It is VLDL with about 4% protein, 8% phospholipid, and 88% neutral fat.

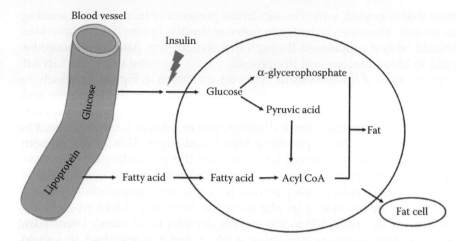

**Figure 10.1** Lipogenesis in fat cells.

surface. During diet or exercise, the sympathetic nerve* secretes noradrenalin,† the adrenal medulla secretes adrenalin, and the anterior pituitary gland secretes adrenocorticotropic hormone,‡ leading to changes in the surface properties of the oil drop so that the lipase can bind with the fat to initiate lipolysis.

## 10.2 Fat synthesis and degradation in the case of obesity

The synthesis and degradation of fat plays a key role in obesity—though, although enzymes degrade fat, the enzyme activity is not necessarily the main factor regulating the reaction. It can be a criterion to decide whether enzymatic reactions in cells are active or low because the presence of active reactions mean increased enzyme synthesis and eventually enhanced enzyme activity.

In the case of an obese person, both the synthesis and degradation of cellular fat are prominent, but the amount of fat synthesized is larger

---

* *Sympathetic nerve*: An area of the central nervous system that controls the function of mobilizing physical resources or energy to quickly respond to an emergency or a stressful situation.

† *Noradrenalin*: A catecholamine hormone secreted from the adrenal medulla, which is also called norepinephrine. Its biologic activity is similar to that of adrenaline but lower than that of adrenaline.

‡ *Adrenocorticotrophic hormone*: A hormone secreted from the pituitary gland to elicit a quick response to stress when felt, which is also delivered to various secretory glands in the body through blood and is thereby involved in the secretion of approximately 30 types of other hormones.

than that degraded, which results in the presence of increased fat, leading to obesity. Therefore, in order to prevent obesity, lipogenesis in lipocytes should be first suppressed through diet structuring. Attention should be paid to blood glucose and lipoprotein, which are substances used in the configuration of lipogenesis in lipocytes, as shown in Figure 10.1.

The problem with glucose is that it cannot enter the lipocytes and take part in lipogenesis without the help of insulin. This is directly shown by the fact that in the case of diabetes, where insulin activity is low, the patient loses weight despite their high blood sugar. This means insulin is not a problem for glucose because even if a person consumes sugar, he/she will not become obese if the insulin level does not rise. Insulin is secreted from β cells of the pancreas in response to stimulation by blood sugar, and the amount of insulin secretion increases 10-fold when blood sugar increases from 100 to 200 mg per deciliter (1/10 liters). Eventually, if sugar of the same calorific value is taken, and it is absorbed, in a short time and the blood sugar level rapidly rises, the person will become obese, but if the sugar is slowly absorbed over a long period and the blood sugar level does not rise significantly, the person will not become obese.

Obesity can be prevented by eating rice in the boiled form without making it into powder because the action of amylase, a starch-hydrolyzing enzyme, will be so low that the starch will be digested slowly and the absorption of the digested starch by the gut will take time. On the other hand, bread that contains a lot of white sugar is quickly absorbed by the action of sucrase, a sugar-hydrolyzing enzyme, so that the blood sugar level rises quickly and the person can easily become obese. When brown sugar is used instead of white sugar, phenyl glucoside (a glycoside resulting from the binding of phenyl and glucose) contained in the black part inhibits the absorption of glucose by the gut, thereby preventing the rapid increase of the blood sugar level so as to help avoid obesity.

Lipoproteins, which are the substrates of lipogenesis in lipocytes, include chylomicron and VLDL. The former contains food-derived fat and the latter contains the fat synthesized in the liver. Therefore, the lipoprotein that can be controlled by diet is chylomicron. When chylomicron comes in contact with lipoprotein, the fatty acid hydrolase binds to heparan sulfate in the endothelial membrane of the blood vessels, the phospholipase A degrades the phospholipid on the surface of chylomicron so that the fat beneath the phospholipid and the lipoprotein fatty acid hydrolase are bound, and degradation begins. The resulting glycerol and fatty acid are mainly metabolized in the liver, but fatty acids enter lipocytes and become fat material. However, not all of the chylomicron-derived fatty acid becomes fat.

The fatty acid formed in the walls of blood vessels of the skeletal muscles enters the muscle cells, where it breaks down into carbonic acid (eventually $CO_2$) and water through β-oxidation (continuous oxidation of carbon atoms at the β site lead to the decomposition of fatty acid into acetyl CoA). The former is discharged through respiration and the latter is excreted out from the body through urine. Eventually, the fat in the meal is metabolized in the skeletal muscles and goes out of the body. However, the fatty acid metabolism in the skeletal muscles differs among different individuals. Fat is actively metabolized in those who exercise daily, whereas the metabolic process is as smooth in those who do not do so adequately. Therefore, abundant metabolism of chylomicron in skeletal muscles is important for preventing obesity. To prevent chylomicron from becoming fat in lipocytes, it is necessary to raise the chylomicron level in the blood rapidly, meaning that the dietary fat should be slowly absorbed, quite similarly in nature to with respect to glucose. However, unlike glucose, which can enter lipocytes only when helped by insulin, chylomicron-derived fatty acids do not require assistance from hormones such as insulin. Ultimately, for obesity prevention, attention should be paid to fatty acids rather than blood glucose. The ratio of fat in South Korean diets has now increased to about 25% today from an amount of only 3% to 5% 50 years ago. The prevalence of obesity is directly proportional to the fat accumulation, and the fat-derived chylomicron in the diet causes obesity.

In order to control obesity, the minimal fat content in diets and its low absorption is very vital to check the rapid rise in the level of chylomicron.

## 10.3   Obesity prevention by chitosan

### 10.3.1   Inhibition of fat absorption in the gut

The fat present in the food is mixed with bile acid* or phospholipid in the duodenum to form small oil globules. Fat is never absorbed as such in the intestine. It is always absorbed after being decomposed into free fatty acids and β-monoglycerides by the pancreatic lipase in the duodenum (Figure 10.2). Fat is not soluble in water, so many fat molecules congregate and form oil droplets. Since the lipase enzyme is water-soluble, the degradation of fat occurs at the interfaces of the oil droplets. Bile acids and phospholipids are present at the interfaces of oil droplets, and are called interfacial active agents.[†] The wider the surface is, the more actively the lipase enzyme acts. In addition to this, bile acid also acts as an activating factor that improves the lipase activity.

The inhibition of either the degradation or absorption process of fat can reduce chylomicron and eventually can prevent the obesity. For instance, the chitosan obtained from crab shells and the chondroitin

---

* *Bile acid*: A steroid acid that is produced from cholesterol in the liver and that helps in fat digestion.
† *Interfacial active agent*: A substance that adheres to the interfaces between a gas and a liquid, between liquids, and between a liquid and a solid in solutions to reduce the interfacial tension.

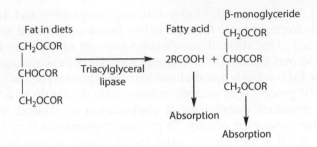

*Figure 10.2* Degradation and absorption of fats in diets.

sulfuric acid* extracted from salmon head region cartilage have been shown to inhibit fat absorption.

To confirm this, Sugano et al. (1978) prepared two types of oil drops using triolein fat and bile acid either with lecithin or gum arabic. In oil drop 1, the bile acid and lecithin exist on the interface around triolein, while in oil drop 2, the bile acid and gum arabic exist on the interface around triolein (Figure 10.3).

Later, a fatty acid-degrading enzyme was applied to the oil drops along with various concentrations of chitosan and chondroitin sulfate. As shown in Figure 10.4, chitosan inhibited the oil drops formed with lecithin but did not inhibit those formed with gum arabic.

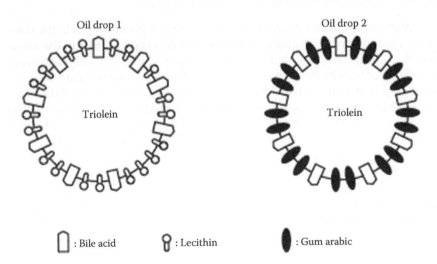

*Figure 10.3* Two types of oil drop formed using lecithin and gum arabic, respectively.

* *Chondroitin sulfate*: A sort of acidic mucopolysaccharide generally distributed in animal connective tissues, centering on cartilage.

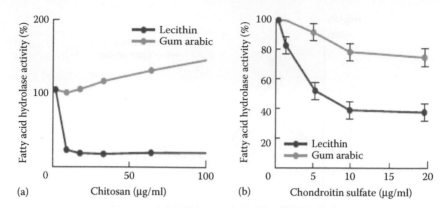

*Figure 10.4* Inhibition of fatty acid hydrolase activity on two types of oil drops by chitosan (a) and chondroitin sulfate (b).

The oil drops formed in the duodenum use lecithin instead of gum arabic. If chitosan acts on the enzyme to inhibit it, the inhibitory action should occur on both oil drops. However, the fact that chitosan inhibited the oil drops formed using lecithin only and did not inhibit others formed using gum arabic emphasizes the idea that chitosan acts on the oil drops rather than on the enzyme to inhibit the reactions.

Glucosamine is a constituent of chitosan and its positively charged amino group forms ionic bonds with negatively charged lecithin to cover the surface of small oil drops, thereby hindering the access of enzyme to inhibit fatty acid degradation.

The action of chondroitin sulfate is different from that of chitosan (Figure 10.4). Chondroitin sulfate not only inhibits the lipase activity on the triolein matrix, containing lecithin but also feebly inhibits that on the triolein matrix, containing gum arabic.

Chondroitin sulfate shows inhibitory activity on the fatty acid hydrolase, thereby deterring its binding to the matrix. This infers that chondroitin sulfate not only inhibits the lipase activity but also inhibits the absorption of the fatty acid resulting from lipolysis in the gut. Although chitosan has shown the prospect to inhibit the absorption of fat in the gut by inhibiting the lipolysis, its role in reducing fat (chylomicron) in blood needs to be evaluated.

In an experiment, 6 mL corn oil, 80 mg bile acid, 2 g cholesterol oliet, and 6 mL water were ultrasonicated thoroughly to make oil drops and were administered to rats. Following administration, the serum fat level was escalated, indicating that the chylomicron level was also increased. Following this, when 1 mL of oil drop and 125 mg chitosan were administered with 1 mL of biological saline solution, the serum neutral fat level significantly dropped (Figures 10.5 and 10.6), indicating

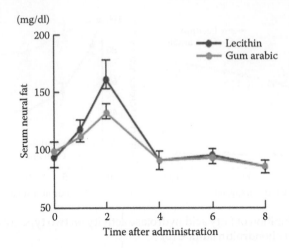

*Figure 10.5* Action of chitosan on serum neutral fat after administration of corn oil.

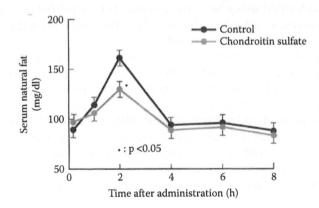

*Figure 10.6* The findings of chondroitin sulfate, which inhibits the lipase activity to subside fatty acid absorption. In this experiment, 1 mL each of oil drop and biological saline solution were orally administered to rats; the results indicated the serum neutral fat level was rapidly increased. However, when 1 mL of a biological saline solution containing 1 mL of oil drops and 20 mg of chondroitin sulfate was administered, the serum neutral fat level was significantly dropped. This proves that chondroitin sulfate inhibited the lipase activity and the absorption of fatty acid, thus blocking the rapid increase of chylomicron.

that chitosan inhibited the rapid upsurge of the chylomicron level through the inhibition of fat absorption.

### 10.3.2 Anti-obesity activity of chitosan and chondroitin sulfate

Chitosan and chondroitin sulfate have shown inhibition of the absorption of dietary fat in the gut to check the prompt increase of fat (chylomicron) in the blood. In a study conducted by Okuda (2001), the role of chitosan was assessed in preventing induced obesity in rats. The rats were supplemented with a high-fat diet containing 400 g of glycerol per kg, or provided control diets instead, for nine weeks. Thereafter, a blood sample was collected and fat tissues around the reproductive organs and the liver were extracted. It was observed that, as a result of high-fat diet administration, the fat tissue weight around the reproductive organs increased as compared with in the controls, leading to obesity. However, the addition of 3%, 7%, or 15% chitosan significantly decreased the fat tissues around the reproductive organs and, hence, averted obesity (Figure 10.7).

The higher fat accumulation led to fatty liver, while the chitosan reduced the fat mass to improve the fatty liver (Figure 10.8).

The increased blood fat was also reduced by chitosan (Figure 10.9).

In this study (Sumiyoshi and Kimura, 2006), it was also revealed that chitosan prevented obesity, fatty liver, and hyperlipidemia from occurring in the rats even after the administration of high-fat diets.

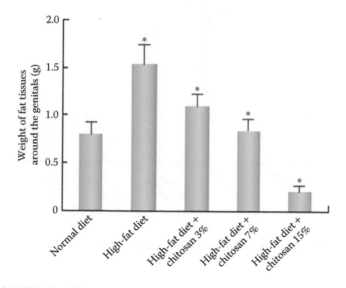

*Figure 10.7* Weight of fat tissues around the genitals.

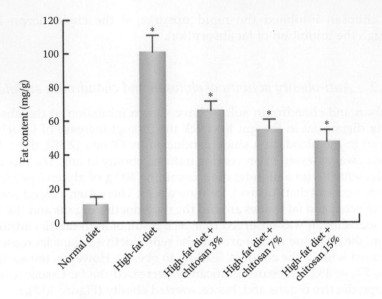

**Figure 10.8** Fat contents in the liver.

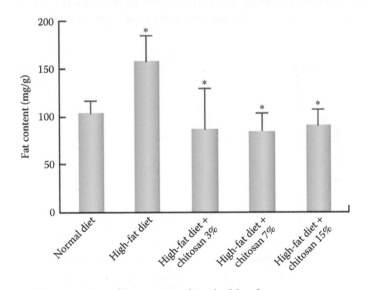

**Figure 10.9** The amounts of fat contained in the blood.

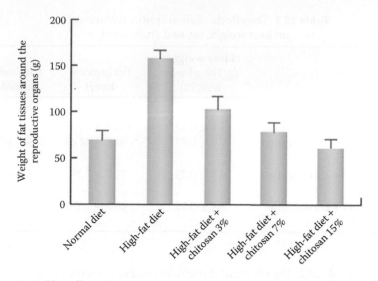

*Figure 10.10* The effect of chondroitin sulfate on the weight of fat tissues around the reproductive organs.

In a very similar experiment, chitosan was replaced with chondroitin sulfate, a similar high-fat diet was administered for eight weeks, and the same parameters were measured. A two-fold increase in fat tissue around the reproductive organs was recorded as compared with in the controls, leading to obesity (Figure 10.10). However, the addition of 7% and 13% chondroitin sulfate drastically decreased the fat tissue weight, indicating the prevention of the obesity induced by high-fat diets.

An increase in liver weight, fat, and cholesterol level induced by high-fat diets can also be controlled by the addition of chondroitin sulfate (Table 10.1). Furthermore, the addition of chondroitin sulfate also inhibits the elevation of the serum fat or cholesterol levels due to the administration of high-fat diets (Table 10.2). These results show the possible role of chondroitin sulfate in preventing obesity, fatty liver, and hyperlipidemia induced by high-fat diets.

Although chitosan and chondroitin sulfate exhibited comparable results and prevented obesity, fatty liver, and hyperlipidemia induced by high-fat diets containing 40% fat and oils, they differ in their mechanisms of action. Chitosan only inhibits the lipolysis, whereas chondroitin sulfate

*Table 10.1* The effects of chondroitin sulfuric acid
on liver weight, fat, and cholesterol

| Division | Liver weight (g/100 g body weight) | Fat (μmol/g liver) | Cholesterol (μmol/g) |
|---|---|---|---|
| Ordinary diet | 5.3 ± 0.15 | 21.2 ± 2.58 | 8.4 ± 0.44 |
| High fat diet | 7.6 ± 0.23 | 124.5 ± 7.73 | 11.7 ± 0.31 |
| High fat diet + chondroitin sulfate 3% | 7.1 ± 0.57 | 94.2 ± 14.64 | 8.8 ± 0.41 |
| High fat diet + chondroitin sulfate 7% | 6.5 ± 0.25 | 72.7 ± 7.19 | 8.3 ± 0.31 |
| High fat diet + chondroitin sulfate 13% | 6.4 ± 0.13 | 68.7 ± 6.16 | 7.6 ± 0.32 |

*Table 10.2* The effects of chondroitin sulfate on serum lipid

| Division | Fat (mM) | Cholesterol (mM) | Free fatty acid (mEq/l) |
|---|---|---|---|
| Ordinary diet | 1.94 ± 0.13 | 1.94 ± 0.11 | 0.66 ± 0.04 |
| High fat diet | 274 ± 0.04 | 2.76 ± 0.15 | 0.98 ± 0.06 |
| High fat diet + chondroitin sulfate 3% | 1.86 ± 0.08 | 2.22 ± 0.12 | 0.90 ± 0.05 |
| High fat diet + chondroitin sulfate 7% | 1.91 ± 0.09 | 2.17 ± 0.15 | 0.86 ± 0.06 |
| High fat diet + chondroitin sulfate 13% | 1.69 ± 0.11 | 1.94 ± 0.08 | 0.82 ± 0.04 |

inhibits both the lipolysis and the absorption of fatty acids, thereby reducing the absorption of beef tallow in the gut to inhibit the rapid rise of chylomicron in the blood.

Chitosan is well-known to lower cholesterol and the neutral fat in the blood due to the fact that it binds with bile acids. Professor Sugano (1980) conducted an experiment and revealed that the binding capacity of chitosan in the acidic region is stronger than that of pectin, which has been known for a long period of time and is similar to that of cholestyramine, which is used as a bile acid-fixing agent.

On daily basis, about 1 g of bile acid is produced from cholesterol in the liver. Meanwhile, bile acid secreted into duodenum amounts to

30 g. The 1 g of bile acid produced in the liver should obviously be insufficient for the secretion of as much as 30 g into the duodenum. Consequently, any bile acid secreted into the duodenum is reabsorbed in the intestine and returned to the liver through the portal vein.* This is called the enterohepatic circulation of bile acid. The amount of bile acid excreted in feces is only 0.8 g. The average cholesterol in diets is 0.5 g, the cholesterol secreted with bile is 2 g, and the cholesterol converted to sterol by the action of intestinal cells excreted in feces is nearly 0.4 g.

If the excretion of bile acid is enhanced by chitosan, more bile acid should be synthesized from cholesterol in the liver. Therefore, as bile acid synthesis progresses, cholesterol level in the blood decreases because it is used as a precursor. Professor Sugano (1978) investigated the effects of chitosan administration in rats for 20 days and revealed that chitosan treatment reduced plasma cholesterol.

## 10.4  Anti-obesity effects of marine algae

Professor Jeon of Jeju National University, South Korea, conducted a study (Kang et al., 2016) to evaluate the anti-obesity properties of different marine algae and identified the inhibitory effects of *Ishige sinicola* and *Gelidium* extracts on pre-adipocyte differentiation and weight gain, which is a fundamental step of the anti-obesity mechanism. The fat accumulated in adipocytes was stained and observed with the naked eyes.

The results as shown in Figure 10.11 indicated that a fewer amount of fat cells were generated in groups treated with *Ishige sinicola* or *Gelidium* extracts, thereby inhibiting the fat accumulation, eventually leading to anti-obesity properties (Figure 10.12).

Studies conducted on the inhibition of differentiation of fat cells mainly use preadipocytes derived from mouse embryos and the differentiation of preadipocytes requires several inducers, such as insulin. The most important steps of differentiation of preadipocytes into fat cells are regulated by peroxisome proliferator-activated receptor γ, cytosine-cytosine-adenosine-adenosine-thymidine-enhancer binding protein α, and sterol regulatory element binding proteins-lc. These transcription factors (TFs) promote the conversion of ingested excessive energy sources into neutral fat, which is stored in fat cells and liver tissues. Therefore, most of

---

* *Portal vein*: A capillary network formed by the branching of veins returning to the heart in the course of returning to the heart.

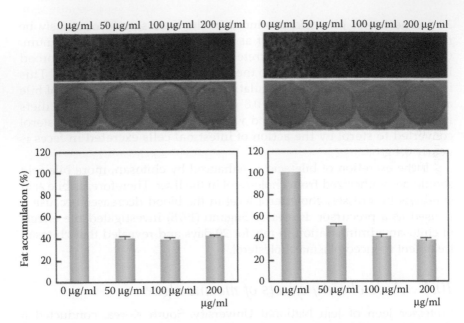

**Figure 10.11** Fat cell differentiation inhibitory effects of *Ishige sinicola* and *Gelidium* extracts.

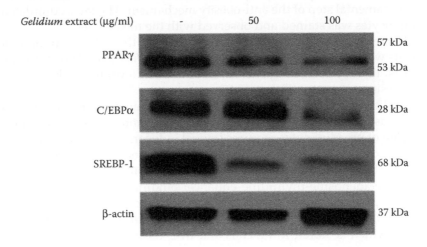

**Figure 10.12** Obesity-inducing factor-controlling efficacy of sea algae extract.

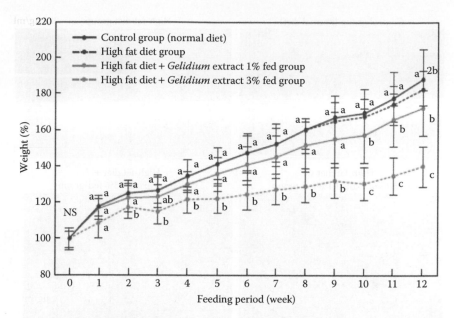

*Figure 10.13* Weight-changing effects of marine algae extracts on an animal obesity model induced by high-fat diets.

the studies to decipher the action mechanism of anti-obesity have been conducted on knocking down the expression of the TFs. As clearly mentioned earlier, *Gelidium* extract inhibits the expression of these three TFs in a dose-dependent manner.

In addition to anti-obesity effects, the oral administration of 1% *Gelidium* extract with high-fat diets for 12 weeks to an obesity model animal did not result in a significant loss in weight, but the use of a higher dose of 3% *Gelidium* extract in the diet was attributed to significant weight reduction (Figure 10.13).

Simultaneously, the microscopic analysis of the fat distribution in fat tissues extracted from an obesity animal model on high-fat diets clearly showed the increase in fat content in the high-fat diet group but a decrease in the diet groups administered with 1% and 3% *Gelidium* extracts. Further, the higher the dose of *Gelidium* extract used, the more prominently the fat content was decreased (Figure 10.14).

Control group (normal diet)          High-fat diet group

High-fat diet +                      High-fat diet +
*Gelidium* extract 1% fed-group      *Gelidium* extract 3% fed-group

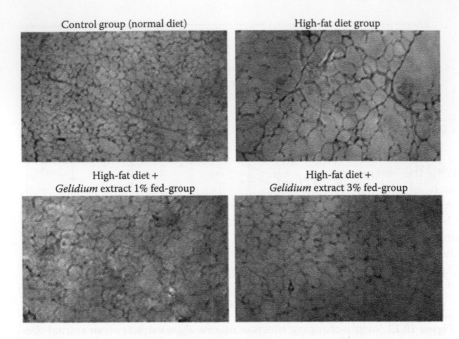

**Figure 10.14** Microscopic analysis of fat distribution in fat cells extracted from animal obesity models induced by high-fat diets.

These results clearly indicate towards the anti-obesity effects of *Gelidium* extract, as it reduced body weight in various model animals. Therefore, *Gelidium* extract has an immense therapeutic potential to be explored as an obesity control agent in the near future.

## chapter eleven

# Osteoporosis and fish bone water-soluble calcium

With the emergence of diverse lifestyle-related diseases and disorders, such as diabetes, hypertension, and arteriosclerosis, and an increase in osteoporosis, South Korea is rapidly becoming an aging society. Osteoporosis is a condition characterized by a reduction in bone mineral and bone matrix and by a change in the microstructure of the bone mass, thereby leading to an increased incidence in fracture cases or in the risk of them. The causes of osteoporosis include a lack of intake of minerals, such as calcium and vitamin D; poor control of physical conditions in females; a decline in estrogen (follicular hormone) secretion due to menopause; and a lack of exercise.

To prevent osteoporosis, an adequate amount of calcium should be included in the diet right from the initial growth phase of the human body so as to reach the maximum bone mass. With respect to preventive measures for osteoporosis, a lack of proper calcium intake has been pointed out as the major problem. In the light of this fact, the intake of calcium exceeding the current nutritional requirement is encouraged and has ignited a surge in the use of calcium supplements.

In recent years, a common problem, especially among junior high school students, is a severe cut-down on healthy food intake in the name of dieting, with an ultimate aim of not becoming plump or obese. However, negligence in the uptake of proper nutrients and vitamins affects the process of bone development and growth. As a result of this, by middle age, the number of osteoporosis patients is expected to increase rapidly. Osteoporosis tests are usually completed when bones are weakened due to the process of aging. In fact, bone health is determined at adolescence, when the bones have reached their peak growth. Currently, the number of patients with osteoporosis in South Korea is approximately 810,000 (Health Insurance Review & Assessment Service, 2013), and this number has been increasing by 5.6% every year.

The American Academy of Pediatrics (AAP) has already announced that bone health in old age depends on how densely the bones are formed during the growth period. The primary factor that threatens and affects bone health is diet. According to the results of the School Health Examination Sample Survey announced by the Ministry of Education in February 2015, five out of every 100 middle- and high-school girls are underweight. The term *underweight* refers to a human with a body mass index (BMI; an individual's body weight divided by the square of their height) of 18.5 or less. Underweighted persons in whom the weight load is not properly distributed on the bones are reported to have approximately a five to six times higher risk of onset of osteoporosis than do people with normal weight.

Osteoporosis in itself is a highly deceptive disorder, owing to the fact that no particular symptoms appear in adolescence despite the presence of weakening bones; however, the situation changes after middle age. If the maximum bone mass (amount of bone) is assumed to be 100, those people who are able to reach a mark only up to 50 in their adolescence cannot exceed it even after the middle age, no matter how strenuous the efforts they make are. The weakening of bones starts from the fifties at a sharp pace such that the bone density decreases by 1% to 2% per year thereafter. This is attributed to an imbalance in the activity of osteoblasts[*] and osteoclasts.[†] Therefore, bone health constitutes an important part of adolescence when osteoblasts are maximally active. During adolescence, bone density is filled steeply until a peak bone mass is reached. Up to 85% of the maximum bone mass is attained by the ages of 21 and 19 years in the case of males and females, respectively. Vitamin D, calcium, growth hormones, and exercises serve as the major factors that stimulate bone growth.

According to the International Osteoporosis Foundation, a 10% increase in the bone density can slow the onset of osteoporosis by 13 years. However, physiological aging of the bones begins in the old age, which is manifested by diverse changes, including a decrease in nutrients and hormone activities that leads to a decrease in bone mass of approximately 2% to 3% per year. These changes are regarded as a syndrome rather than a disease and can be prevented or treated to some extent in some cases.

Bone tissue consists of bone matrixes and bone salts (hydroxyapatite crystals in the bone matrix of collagen fibers), collectively known as bone mass. Their ratio remains constant and does not change. Osteoporosis is a condition in which the entire bone mass is in a state of diminution. In contrast, another related condition, called osteomalacia is characterized by ossifluence in which only bone salts decrease due to disorders in bone calcification.

---

[*] *Osteoblast*: A cell that synthesizes and secretes the bone matrix and deposits inorganic salts such as calcium, magnesium, and ions on the matrix to calcify the bone tissue.
[†] *Osteoclast*: A large cell that serves a function of absorbing bone tissues.

The minerals constantly decrease, leading to the thinning and weakening of cartilage, consequently leading to a reduction in the quantity and size of the trabeculae of bones and bone weakening.

Calcium is the only nutrient that is not sufficient to meet the requirement. To improve the calcium deficiency, measures should be taken not only to increase the calcium intake but also to facilitate the process of its absorption and to enhance the rate of its utilization. Compounds that function to enhance calcium absorption and utilization in the body include organic acids, such as citric acid and malic acid; vitamin D; milk sugar; and casein phosphopeptide (CPP).

Conversely, factors that inhibit calcium absorption include oxalic acid (cocoa); phytic acid (cereals, pulses); sulfur-containing amino acids (cysteine, methionine) present in animal proteins; plant fibers; alcohols; and caffeine. The excessive intake of table salt also diminishes calcium absorption. Efforts should aim at maximally utilizing calcium in the living body by considering the above-mentioned positive and negative factors. However, the intake of large amounts of calcium alone may lead to constipation, intestinal edema, and a remarkable decline in the use of iron and zinc in the living body, indicating that the uptake and utilization need to be balanced.

While the United States National Institutes of Health recommends a maximum calcium intake of 1,500 mg per day for all elderly people, an intake of more than 2,000 mg per day may cause side effects. However, considering that having a balance in calcium's intake and utilization is more important than intake quantity, the Japanese *diet intake standard* has determined the maximum allowable limit of calcium intake to be 2,500 mg per day (Table 11.1).

In South Korea, the recommended daily intake of calcium is 700 mg per day; 800 to 900 mg during puberty, a period in which the body grows fast; and 1,000 mg for pregnant women. The calcium that enters the body in the form of food is solubilized in the stomach by various acids present in the stomach, after which it is absorbed in the small intestine. The absorption of calcium is highly pH-dependent and therefore, for maximum absorption, calcium should be present in a water-soluble state in

*Table 11.1* Calcium intake ratios by food group

| Type | Internal resorption rate (%) |
| --- | --- |
| Anchovy, sardine | 20 ~ 30 |
| Milk | 50 ~ 60 |
| Marine algae | 4.5 |
| Vegetables | 18 |
| Cereals and potatoes | 6.1 |

the intestine since the pH of the small intestine is neutral. For instance, milk, which contains calcium, is known to be absorbed well because the calcium in it is present in an aqueous state in neutral pH.

With regard to the above-mentioned calcium deficiency frequently observed, especially among youngsters, and the increasing incidence of osteoporosis, the effective use of massively abandoned fish bones is important both for improving environmental contamination by its disposal and in serving as an alternative calcium source. With this background, Kato et al. (2001) investigated the effects of calcium phosphate and fish bone calcium, which are used as calcium agents, on bone functions and composition to review the effectiveness of fish bones as a calcium source and to study the amount of calcium intake necessary during the growth periods of experimental animals.

Kato et al., in their 1994 study, fed male rats during the growth period with a diet containing calcium in the form of calcium phosphate, salmon bone powder, and yellow tail bone powder in a range of 0 and 2,000 mg per 2,000 kcal for a period of six weeks, and subsequently investigated changes in the weight of the rats. According to the results, the samples that did not contain calcium adversely affected growth and development by suppressing weight gain as compared with in the groups fed on a diet containing calcium. However, there was almost no difference in the weight gains made due to differences in the calcium sources.

These results highlight the fact that calcium is not only involved in bone formation but is also required for proper growth and development. Although 99% of calcium is present in the bones and teeth, the remaining 1% is present in the muscles and blood, which constitutes a very small amount, and is involved in various biocontrol systems, such as neurotransmission, muscle contraction, energy generation, blood coagulation, and the activation of enzymes involved in metabolism.

In the calcium phosphate diet group, bone strength increased in proportion to calcium contents up to the level of 1,200 mg per 2,000 kcal. However, no change was observed with respect to higher calcium contents. The salmon and yellowtail bone calcium groups exhibited similar results to the calcium phosphate group in terms of bone strength, suggesting that fish bones that could not be easily utilized as food materials until now can be easily harvested to be utilized as effective calcium sources. Although the bone strength increased in proportion to the amount of calcium intake, no difference in the weight of the bones was observed. It was observed, however, that the bone strength decreased when the amount of calcium intake was low, due to an increase in the amount of water that resulted from a decrease in the amount of bone minerals. Upon investigation of a correlation between bone strength and composition, the correlation was found to be prominent at calcium content levels of lower than 1,000 mg. Moreover, there was a little change at higher calcium contents, eventually indicating that the minimum amount of calcium necessary to maintain bone metabolism is approximately 1,200 mg.

Regarding the uptake of calcium by the gut, the calcium absorption rate was high, amounting to approximately 80% when the amount of calcium phosphate intake was up to 1,200 mg. However, it decreased when the amount of calcium phosphate intake was higher than 1,200 mg. Also, an excessive intake led to a reduction in the calcium absorption rate, implying that a control system that prevents the absorption of excessive calcium in the body was operating. From the results in terms of absorption, the required amount of calcium was estimated to be approximately 1,200 mg. The fish bone calcium was considered usable for the bones because the resultant strength was not different, although the absorption rate was low.

## 11.1   Iron metabolism and calcium

Massive intake of calcium phosphate or calcium carbonate has been shown to inhibit the absorption of non-heme iron (iron that binds in non-heme states in iron-containing proteins). In adult women, iron-deficiency anemia, like osteoporosis, is a major problem.

Kato (2001) investigated the effects of differences in calcium sources on iron absorption using fish bone calcium and calcium phosphate. The group used male rats in the growth period as the experimental animals and rats after resecting two-thirds of the liver, which is involved in the metabolism of minerals such as calcium and iron. These were compared with normal rats (control).

The liver is an organ that activates the vitamin D necessary for the absorption of calcium. It also serves as a reservoir of iron. The effects of different sources of calcium on the use of iron in the living body were examined in detail using rats with the quantity of iron in storage reduced by liver resection. The calcium sources used were calcium phosphate and yellow tail bone calcium. The rats were fed on diets with the necessary calcium content of 1,000 mg per 2,000 kcal and on diets with an excessive calcium content of 3,000 mg. These were administered respectively for three weeks. Unfortunately, the bones were not strengthened even after increasing the amount of calcium intake by more than 1,000 mg.

This finding indicated that 1,000 mg of calcium per 2,000 kcal refers to an amount of calcium that is sufficient to maintain bone strength. Also, no difference was observed between the two calcium sources of fish bone calcium and calcium phosphate used. In addition, since the bone strength was maintained and the calcium absorption rate did not change even in rats where most of the liver, which is involved in the activation of vitamin D, was resected, it was assumed that the amount of vitamin D necessary for calcium absorption could be activated only if one-third of the liver remains. A decrease in the rate of absorption of iron in the gut to half was observed, when the amount of calcium in calcium phosphate was increased. However, no iron absorption-suppressing activity appeared even when large amounts of calcium in yellow tail bone powder were ingested. Therefore, it was reported that the calcium in fish bone powder could be an excellent calcium source that would not adversely affect the absorption of iron.

## 11.2   *Physiological effect of fish bones*

The increase in osteoporosis with aging is related to menopause. Previous studies have shown that when estrogen secretion, which is involved in bone formation, decreased or disappeared, the bone mass did not change; however, the body weight increased. To investigate weight change and bone strength using fish bone calcium diets and calcium phosphate diets for a long period of time by resecting the ovaries of mature female rats that had stopped growing, 15-week-old female rats were utilized. Both ovaries from half of them were removed (ovax) and sham operations were performed on the remaining half (sham control). In addition, the rats were divided into two groups; one group was reared with 600 mg/2,000 kcal of calcium phosphate diets, whereas the other group was reared with 600 mg/2,000 kcal of fish bone calcium diets, each for approximately 12 weeks. According to the results, when the ovaries were resected, a compensatory increase in the body fat and weight occurred, but no weight gain was recognized in the rats administered with fish bones. Furthermore, the ovariectomy and differences in calcium source did not affect the bone strength, though the strength of the bones that support the body was reduced by ovariectomy when converted into bone strength per unit weight. However, weight gains were suppressed when fish bones were ingested so that the bone strength per unit weight was recovered to the same level as that of the rats in the sham control group.

The serum neutral fat obtained from ovariectomy was significantly reduced by fish bone intake. Also, the lipoprotein, very low-density lipoprotein (VLDL), which transports the neutral lipid synthesized in the liver to other tissues, was reduced upon intake of fish bone. Although the total cholesterol level in blood increased due to ovariectomy, it was inhibited in the group reared on fish bone calcium intake. Fishbone calcium is effective for the prevention of osteoporosis indirectly because it suppresses unnecessary weight gains, unlike calcium phosphate. Highly unfavorable fatty acids, eicosapentaenoic acid (EPA) and docosahexaenoic acid (DHA), contained in fish bones are effective for improving lipid metabolism. Therefore, fish bone can be said to be not only a calcium source but also a functional nutrition source with added value.

## 11.3   Fish fat (fat-soluble vitamin) and osteoporosis

In addition to the nutritional values that have been discovered, vitamins have physiological actions that contribute to the prevention of cancer and diseases related with lifestyle. Therefore, these are gaining attention as functional substances and nutrients. In addition to the highly unsaturated fatty acids,[*] EPA and DHA, fish oils contain large amounts of lipid-soluble vitamins, which are advantageous to food functionalities derived from seafood processing byproducts. In particular, the prevention of osteoporosis in elderly persons by the intake of vitamin D from fish oils may greatly contribute to the maintenance and improvement of health in elderly people.

The distribution of fat-soluble vitamins (A, D, and E) in fishes can be reviewed by using the example of carp, which is a representative freshwater fish. The hepatopancreas contains the largest amount of vitamin A per unit weight, followed by orbital[†] fat, red color meat, and white color meat, in order of precedence. Orbital fat and the hepatopancreas contain the largest amount of vitamin D per unit weight, followed by red and white color meat, respectively, in order of precedence. Like vitamin D, orbital fat contains the largest amount of vitamin E. Red color meat also contains some vitamin E; however, white color meat and hepatopancreas contain little vitamin E. In this respect, the orbital fat and hepatopancreas of carp can be said to be useful sources of fat-soluble vitamins.

As for the distribution of fat-soluble vitamins (A, D, and E) in tuna, which is a seawater fish, the liver contains the largest amount of vitamin A per unit weight, followed by red color meat, orbital fat, heart, and white color meat, in order of precedence. The orbital fat and liver contain the largest amounts of vitamin D, followed by the heart, red color meat, and white color meat. Similarly, the orbital fat contains the largest amount of vitamin E, followed by the liver and white color meat. Although the distribution of

---

[*] *Highly unsaturated fatty acid*: Highly unsaturated fatty acids having four or more double bonds.
[†] *Orbital*: A space in the skull that contains the eyeball. It is surrounded by bones and contains muscles around the eyes, blood vessels, and nerves.

fat-soluble vitamins in tuna is similar to that of carp, vitamin E is not present in the orbital fat of tuna, though a large amount of it is contained in the liver. When seen relatively, the fat-soluble vitamin contents of tuna are higher than those of carp. Therefore, active and effective intake of vitamins and biofactors (living body substances that are indispensable for living organisms to carry out basic functions, although they are only needed in small quantities) of marine products are expected to have the ability to not only prevent osteoporosis or rickets but also to treat cancers and autoimmune diseases. When strictly defined, vitamin D can be better called a lipid biofactor synthesized from 7-dehydroxycholesterol in human skin epithelium. However, the requirement cannot be sufficiently met with only the foregoing synthesis; more vitamin D should be ingested through proper diet.

## 11.4  Effects of fish oil on calcium absorption and bone formation

It has already been shown that vitamin D is important for bone formation and involved in the actions of bones and diseases such as osteoporosis. The orbital fat of fish has been described as a useful source of vitamin D. Also, the contents of vitamin D are generally higher in larger fishes.

The calcium absorption rate, amount of retained calcium, and net calcium utilization rate of rats (fish oil diet group) who ingested feeds containing tuna orbital fat with high vitamin D contents as a lipid source (lipid content: 25%, calcium content: 4,776 mg/1,000 g, vitamin D content: 504,695 IU/1,000 g) were compared with those of rats (beef tallow diet group) who ingested feeds containing beef tallow as a lipid source (lipid content: 25%, calcium content: 4,774 mg/1,000 g, vitamin D content: 2,330 IU/1,000 g). Although the calcium absorption rate of the fish oil diet group was higher than that of the beef tallow diet group, the calcium retention rate was high in both of the groups and displayed no intergroup differences. Therefore, when the difference in calcium absorption rates was reflected, the net calcium utilization rate of the fish oil diet group was higher than that of the beef tallow diet group.

When rats were reared using feeds mixed with fish oil and beef tallow, respectively, the body weight gains of the two groups were almost the same as each other during the entire rearing period. When the rearing was finished, weights increased to approximately 1.5 times to those when the rearing was initiated. The dry weights of the femurs extracted after the rearing were higher in rats reared with feeds containing larger amounts of fish oil.

In addition, the bone strength of rats was found to increase as the amount of fish oil contained in the feed increased. Moreover, calcium concentration generally tended to increase as the amount of fish oil contained in the feed increased.

These results suggest that fish orbital fat is a useful source of vitamin D and is beneficial for the prevention of osteoporosis, a cause of vitamin D deficiency, and for the maintenance of the bone density.

## 11.5   Development of water-soluble calcium from fish bones

Taking into consideration the fact that large fishes can easily degrade the bones of small fishes when they prey on them, we extracted crude enzymes from fish guts and decomposed fish bones using the crude enzymes to prepare water-soluble calcium.

When the water-soluble calcium agent prepared was administered to rats with osteoporosis, the strength of the femur increased to a similar extent as that seen when the milk-derived calcium absorption enhancer (CPP) was administered (Figure 11.1).

The amount of calcium that was introduced into musculoskeletal cells after the administration of water-soluble calcium was also similar to that when CPP was administered (Figure 11.2).

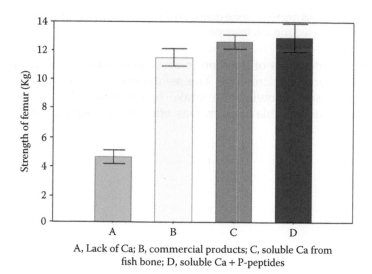

A, Lack of Ca; B, commercial products; C, soluble Ca from fish bone; D, soluble Ca + P-peptides

*Figure 11.1* Measurement of the femur strength of experimental rats.

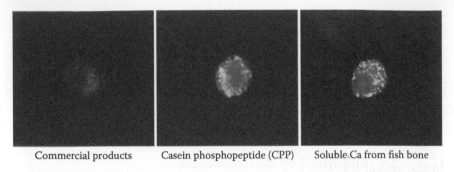

Commercial products      Casein phosphopeptide (CPP)      Soluble Ca from fish bone

*Figure 11.2* Calcium absorption effect in osteoblasts after treatment with water-soluble calcium.

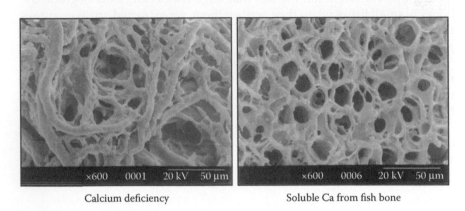

Calcium deficiency                    Soluble Ca from fish bone

*Figure 11.3* A cross-section (bone density) of the femur of an experimental rat as seen through an electron microscope.

The bone densities of the femurs of experimental rats were checked through an electron microscope. The results demonstrated that the bone density increased following the intake of water-soluble calcium, indicating that water-soluble calcium was effective in treating osteoporosis (Figure 11.3).

# chapter twelve

# Sexual dysfunction
## Impotence and Urechis unicinctus

In the sexual life, if one or more conditions such as erection, pleasure, duration, ejaculation, and relaxation do not occur, the phenomenon is called a sexual dysfunction. A condition in which insertion is impossible in 75% or more cases of sexual intercourse with symptoms persisting for at least three months is called impotence.

Upon reviewing recent impotence prevalence rates, it can be seen that the United States exhibits the highest rate of and Japan shows the lowest rate of impotence at 52% and 28%, respectively, indicating that impotence is a problem worldwide (Figure 12.1).

In the case of South Korea, the impotence prevalence rates above slight impotence are 23% in the thirties, 34% in the forties, 64% in the fifties, and 86% in the sixties or older ages, indicating a pattern of increase in proportion with increasing age (Figure 12.2).

Nevertheless, the phenomenon of impotence has been accepted or abandoned naturally as a phenomenon resulting from aging rather than a disease in many cases. However, recently, impotence has been considered very important in terms of quality of life. It is increasingly becoming a perception that it is a disease that needs to be treated.

The purpose of the treatment of impotence is to ensure that the individual or the partner has satisfactory instances of sexual intercourse. For this, the cause of impotence needs to be established to bring about desired changes in lifestyle or risk factors so that a desirable sexual life can be achieved. In addition, impotence is associated with other risk factors for cardiovascular system diseases, such as diabetes, hypertension, and hyperlipidemia. Therefore, the fact that impotence may appear as a premonitory symptom of more serious medical diseases, such as diabetes or hypertension, should always be kept in mind.

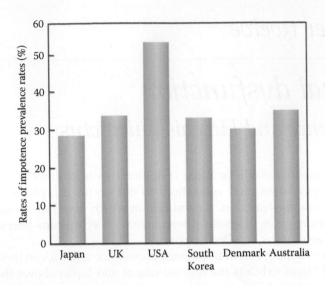

**Figure 12.1** Impotence prevalence rates by country. (From National Information Portal.)

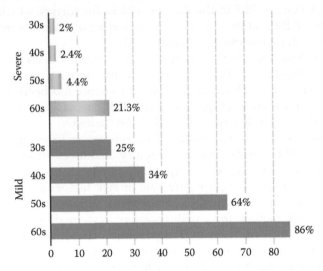

**Figure 12.2** Impotence prevalence rates by country by age and by the degree of symptoms.

## 12.1 Cause of impotence

For the penis to become erect, the blood vessels in the penis must dilate. As shown in Figure 12.3, nitric oxide (NO) is produced from arginine, which is an amino acid, by nitric oxide synthase (NOS). NO, in turn,

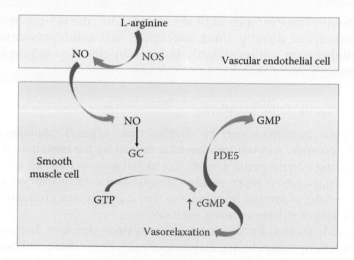

**Figure 12.3** Normal erection mechanism.

plays an important role in erection. When the yield of NO from the vascular endothelial cells increases, it permeates into the smooth muscle cells of the blood vessels to activate the guanylate cyclase,* thereby converting guanosine triphosphate (GTP) into cyclic guanosine monophosphate (cGMP), which leads to the relaxation of the blood vessels. The relaxation of the blood vessels enhances the amount of blood flow while preventing the incoming blood from exiting so that the erection can be maintained (Figure 12.3).

NO, NOS, phosphodiesterase type 5 (PDE5), guanosine monophosphate (GMP), cGMP, GTP, and guanylate cyclase (GC) are the main compounds that participate in the erection.

Although most of the causes of impotence in the past were regarded to be psychogenic and organic causes were regarded as limited to being present only in some cases, recently, organic causes have been found to be more common.

## 12.1.1 Psychogenic impotence

Psychogenic impotence is closely related with anxiety about sexual intercourse, tension, and stressors stemming from the relationship with the partner, especially depression and anxiety. Major symptoms of depression include persistent mood deterioration, loss of interest and pleasure, irregular sleep patterns and appetite, and decreased

---

* *Guanylate cyclase*: An enzyme that catalyzes the formation of cyclic GMP and pyrophosphoric acid using GTP as a substrate.

sexual desire. The dysfunction of the neuroendocrine system observed in depression can directly affect impotence, and antidepressants used to treat depression can secondarily induce impotence or aggravate the symptoms.

## 12.1.2   Vasculogenic impotence

Vasculogenic impotence can be divided into arterial impotence and venous impotence. Arterial impotence is caused by the obstruction of the blood flowing into the penis arteries due to a disease or damage occurring in the penis arteries. A representative disease is coronary arteriosclerosis. A characteristic of arterial impotence is that it progresses gradually, leading to the loss of stiffness during erection.

The risk factors for cardiovascular system diseases include age, hypertension, hyperlipidemia, diabetes, obesity, depression, and excessive smoking. Among these, hyperlipidemia and smoking directly affect the cavernous body of the penis, which is involved in erection. The incidence rates of heart diseases and impotence are proportional to age, implying that damage to the arteries or cavernosal endothelium of the penis and cardiovascular damage can occur simultaneously. Hyperlipidemia inhibits nitrogen monoxide synthase (inducible NOS), leading to impotence, a finding that is in accordance with the fact that hyperlipidemia accompanies 42.4% of patients with impotence.

The use of antihypertensives, such as diuretics, also results in the development of impotence. In patients with diabetes, the hardening of the penis arteries, proliferation of the endothelium due to hyperlipidemia, calcification, and adhesion of the bone occur, resulting in arterial impotence. In smokers, the absorption of nicotine interferes with the relaxation of the penis arteries and the cavernous body, thereby obstructing the flow of blood both in the arteries and in the veins, consequently resulting in impotence.

Venous occlusive impotence occurs when the outflow of the blood through the veins from the cavernous body of the penis is greater than the inflow of the blood through the arteries. A normal erection depends on the flow of blood through the arteries, relaxation of the smooth muscles of the cavernous body of the penis, and functions of Albuginea.* If any of these three functions fail to work normally, the venous occlusive function, which prevents the blood in the cavernous body of the penis from escaping into the systemic vascular system, may be lost, resulting in venous occlusive erectile impotence.

---

* *Albuginea*: A sturdy white layer formed of fibrous tissues that covers the film layer of organs.

## 12.1.3  Neurogenic impotence

Since the neurovascular system of the body is responsible for regulating the erection, disorders or diseases of the brain, spinal cord, cavernosal nerve, or external pudendal nerves can lead to impotence. In addition, many neurological diseases may impair the sensory-cognitive and ejaculatory functions separately from negatively affecting the erectile capacity. The impairment of the central nerves for penis erection can also cause some psychogenic impotence. Neurogenic impotence is caused by brain diseases, such as brain hemorrhage, stroke, and Parkinson's disease, or chronic diseases such as diabetes.

## 12.1.4  Endocrine impotence

A reduction in the level of the male hormone testosterone is manifested by a decline in sexual interest or function. Testosterone increases sexual interest, the frequency of sexual behavior, and the frequency of nocturnal erections. When the level of the male hormone drops, in addition to a decline in the erectile function, the frequency of sexual thoughts or sexual intercourse decreases. It is also accompanied by a decrease in the amount of ejaculatory fluid and by the deterioration of semen properties.

## 12.2  Prevention of impotence by changes in lifestyle

The most basic treatment for impotence is to identify and eliminate the corrective risk factors. In this regard, changes in lifestyle can very effectively reduce the incidence of impotence. Moreover, appropriate drug treatment or psychiatric help is efficient and is known to be quite effective for treating impotence presenting due to psychological causes, in particular. In addition, patients suffering from impotence or erectile dysfunction who also have severe medical diseases, such as diabetes and hypertension, can improve the situation by improving the conditions of their diseases.

Among those individuals who appropriate exercise in mid-life as compared with other long-term solutions, a significant reduction in the incidence of impotence has been observed. In addition, a report indicates that impotence conditions among obese persons could be improved through the performance of intensive exercise for two years. The resultant weight loss and the degree of improvement were related with the intensity of exercise.

Another report indicated that actively reducing body fat resulted in an improvement in impotence conditions within three months. Moreover, a reduction in body fat effectively benefited the patients in whom oral drugs proved to be ineffective in several studies. Although more studies are necessary, the effects of exercise, weight loss, and fat reduction on impotence can serve as strong motivators for lifestyle changes. It is also known that general health problems, sexual dysfunction of the spouse, and the absence of a sex life for a long period of time may lead to disorders in erection, stress, and depression.

Therefore, maintaining the health with a good lifestyle and proper exercise, continuing a healthy sex life, avoiding excessive stress, and maintaining a positive psychological state are indispensable for maintaining the erectile capacity or for recovery from impotence. In addition, having a low-fat diet and eating meals rich in proteins and vitamins and refraining from drinking and smoking are also considered to be important.

## 12.3   Side effects of impotency drugs

The fact that impotency drugs possess a mechanism to increase the arterial blood in the cavernous body of the penis to induce smooth muscle relaxation and penis erection has already been explained. Currently, five PDE5* inhibitors are available in South Korea: Viagra® (component name: sildenafil; Pfizer, New York, NY, USA), Cialis (component name: tadalafil; Eli Lilly and Company, Indianapolis, IN, USA), Levitra (component name: vardenafil; Bayer HealthCare Pharmaceuticals LLC, Berlin, Germany), Zydena (component name: udenafil; Dong-A Pharmaceutical South Korea), and Mvix (component name: mirodenafil; SK Chemicals Life Science, South Korea). These drugs have been proven to be both stable and efficient in treating general impotence and impotence in combinations with special conditions, such as diabetes or prostatectomy. One thing to keep in mind while taking these drugs is that PDE5 inhibitors are not inducers of erection and require sexual stimulation to induce an erection.

PDE5 inhibitors should be taken when a sufficient period of time has passed after eating because of their extensive interactions with food, especially with food rich in fat. However, these interactions are not observed with a small amount of drinking. A study by Porst et al. (2001) reports that most PDE5 inhibitors exhibited sexual intercourse success rates of approximately 75%, with a lower effect in patients with diabetes (50%–55%) or patients who underwent prostatectomy (37%–41%). Studies could hardly compare the usefulness of individual drugs directly due to differences in the selection criteria of individual subject patients. However, there have been reports indicating that these drugs aggravated heart diseases or caused hypotension leading to death in severe patients suffering from a heart disease such as angina or in those who were taking nitrate drugs. Therefore, to prevent such problems, it is desirable to consult a physician and undergo basic cardiovascular system tests before taking one of these drugs.

---

* *Phosphodiesterase type 5*: An enzyme that catalyzes the reaction through which phosphodiester becomes phosphomonoester and alcohol, which is a sort of phosphatase.

These drugs also exhibit side effects, the most common of which is a headache that occurs in approximately 15% of cases. A headache can occur when taking these medications due to the dilatation of blood vessels innervating the brain. In addition, facial flushing, nasal congestion, and dizziness can present in 2% to 10% of cases. However, in the case of Viagra®, cyanopsia (dysopsia under which all objects are seen in blue) or other visual disturbances may appear in rare cases due to the simultaneous inhibition of PDE type 6 present in the retina. In the case of Cialis, low back pain has been rarely reported due to the inhibition of PDE type 11.

Viagra®, while dilating the blood vessels of the penis, tends to dilate blood vessels in other organs too. For instance, if Viagra® affects the dilatation of blood vessels related to the cardiovascular system, patients, especially those suffering from cardiovascular system diseases, should be analyzed for the ability of their heart to cover the quantity of motions for sexual intercourse.

## 12.4   Sexual function improving effects using marine organisms

The Chinese ancient medical book *Chinese Bencao* (*Chinese Herbal Materia Medica*; 中華本草) indicates that more than 180 species of marine living organisms were used as medicinal ingredients. However, only approximately 10 species are presently used, including seahorses, sea dragons, sea cucumbers, starfish, shark cartilage, shellfish, squid bone, and sea algae such as *Sargassum horneri*.

According to *Chinese Bencao* and *Donguibogam* (*Principles and Practice of Eastern Medicine*, Korea), seahorse invigorates men and strengthens virility. Especially in China, seahorses are sold at very high prices as a sexual enhancer at herbal medicine shops and are stored in liquor bottles so that the liquor may be drank like ginseng wine. However, no data or concrete study or clinical test results regarding the claims can be found. Therefore, we studied the effects of seahorses cultured in China on virility to identify two new substances that have similar functions to those of the male hormone androgen.

However, it was difficult to continue studies on the utilization of seahorse in South Korea because these are not cultured in South Korea, and the number of seahorses living in the sea is very small. Therefore, we searched for materials to improve sexual function from various marine living organisms.

NO activates an enzyme called guanylate cyclase to change GTP into cGMP. Since cGMP is a substance that directly induces an erection, NO obtained from diverse marine life species was compared and the results displayed high yields in oyster, scallop, and squid. *Urechis unicinctus*

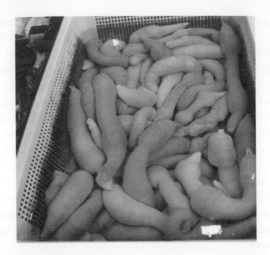

***Figure 12.4*** Picture of *Urechis unicinctus*. (From https://upload.wikimedia. org/wikipedia/commons/7/76/Gaebul.jpg.)

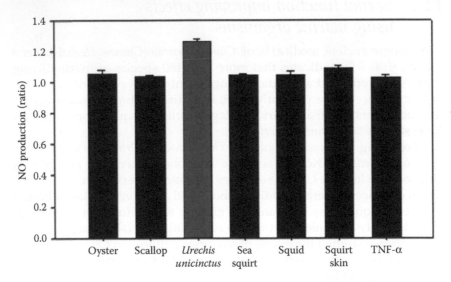

***Figure 12.5*** A comparison of NO yields among diverse marine organisms.

(Figure 12.4) exhibited relatively high NO yields. In particular, the highest NO yield was identified in *U. unicinctus* (Figure 12.5).

The effects of *U. unicinctus* extract on the production of NO and the male hormone testosterone, which are important factors in sexual activity, were checked. The results indicated that the yields of NO and testosterone increased in a *U. unicinctus* extract in a concentration-dependent manner (Figure 12.6).

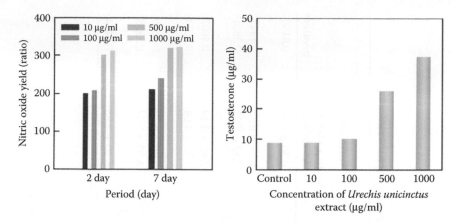

**Figure 12.6** NO and testosterone yields of high temperature/high pressure hot water extracts of *Urechis unicinctus*.

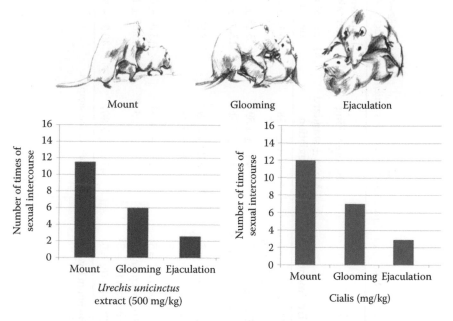

**Figure 12.7** Sexual function improving effects of *Urechis unicinctus* extract (500 mg/kg) and Cialis in animal experiments (measurement of the numbers of times of glooming, mounts, and ejaculations in instances of sexual intercourse).

The efficacy of *U. unicinctus* extract was compared with that of an available drug (Cialis) through animal experiments as shown in Figure 12.6. The results demonstrated that treatment with *U. unicinctus* extract exhibited a similar efficacy to that of Cialis (Figure 12.7). Clinical tests were conducted to identify the efficacy of *U. unicinctus* extract on human bodies.

Table 12.1 Results of clinical tests of *Urechis unicinctus* extract's sexual function improvement

| Treatment group | Before taking | Eight weeks after taking | Variation | p-value[a] |
|---|---|---|---|---|
| | Mean ± standard deviation | Mean ± standard deviation | Mean ± standard deviation | |
| Total testosterone variation | | | | |
| *Urechis unicinctus* extract (N = 3) | 3.11 ± 1.58 | 3.41 ± 0.56 | 0.30 ± 1.96 | 0.8153 |
| Placebo (N = 5) | 4.17 ± 1.59 | 3.58 ± 1.28 | −0.59 ± 0.73 | 0.1447 |
| International index of erectile function | | | | |
| *Urechis unicinctus* extract (N = 3) | 8.67 ± 7.51 | 13.33 ± 3.06 | 4.67 ± 7.23 | 0.3801 |
| Placebo (N = 5) | 16.20 ± 7.69 | 18.80 ± 10.85 | 2.60 ± 6.19 | 0.4007 |
| International prostate symptom score | | | | |
| *Urechis unicinctus* extract (N = 3) | 6.67 ± 4.04 | 5.33 ± 4.04 | 1.33 ± 4.04 | 0.6254 |
| Placebo (N = 5) | 15.4 ± 10.64 | 13.00 ± 6.32 | 2.40 ± 6.73 | 0.4699 |
| Aging male's symptom score | | | | |
| *Urechis unicinctus* extract (N = 3) | 51.67 ± 5.03 | 43.67 ± 14.36 | 8.00 ± 9.54 | 0.2835 |
| Placebo (N = 5) | 45.60 ± 7.80 | 40.20 ± 9.18 | 5.40 ± 8.88 | 0.2454 |

[a] p-value: The significant minimum level in the resultant values of the samples.

In these tests, when the test product (*U. unicinctus* extract) was taken for eight weeks, blood testosterone and liver function values; degrees of impotence; physical improvement (erectile capacity index, prostate symptom); and male climacteric symptom scores by area were observed to improve. Moreover, subjective questionnaire survey results from test subjects indicated that the subjects were satisfied with respect to an improvement in symptoms (Table 12.1).

The extract of *U. unicinctus*, which is a marine living organism, is a natural product without any side effect and is expected to provide hope to men with impotence. The ironic fact is that Japan has the lowest impotence prevalence in the world, as Japanese eat the largest quantity of marine products in the world.

# chapter thirteen

# Sleep disorders and blue mussel extract

The Sleep Dynamics Center at the Catholic University of Korea surveyed and studied the actual states of insomnia and sleep disorders in a national population of 2,375 men and women aged ≥15 years (Park et al., 2007). The results indicated that approximately four million people, representing 12% of the general population, were experiencing insomnia to such extent that they were unable to sleep at night at least three times a week. Insomnia symptoms can be of the following types:

- Insomnia symptoms causing difficulties in sleep appeared in 2.3% of the general population.
- Insomnia symptoms causing frequent awakening after falling into sleep appeared in 8.3% of the general population.
- Insomnia symptoms causing awakening at dawn and difficulties in falling asleep again appeared in 1% of the general population.
- Insomnia symptoms causing nonrestorative sleep that makes the sleeper feel as if he/she did not sleep appeared in 5.1% of the general population.
- Insomnia symptoms causing unsatisfactory sleep appeared in 6.1% of the general population.

All these indicated that sleep disorders are serious health problems. The analytical studies of daytime symptoms in individuals who did not sleep sufficiently showed that 8.3% of them slept for less than five hours a day, in general. As compared with individuals who slept for at least seven hours a day, the individuals sleeping for less than five hours a day showed more daytime sleepiness (4.7 times), fatigue (8.5 times), problems in cognitive functions (6.6 times), mood variations, anxiety and depression (5.7 times), insomnia (6.2 times), and sleep apnea (3.1 times). Sleep is necessary not just for rest because during sleep, brain waves frequently change and important processes such as energy generation and memory enhancement occur. Physical and mental health can be maintained only when these processes progress smoothly. According to the changes observed in brain waves and those occurring in the human body during sleep, sleep is broadly divided into rapid eye movement (REM) sleep and non-REM sleep.

Non-REM sleep is further divided into three stages, depending on the length of sleep.

- *Non-REM sleep stage 1 (process to fall asleep)*: This is a stage in between a sleeping state and the state of being awake, which is maintained for the first 10 minutes after falling asleep. Awakening from sleep because of a feeling of falling from a height or an observation of flashing lights mainly occurs at this stage. The feeling of having had sound sleep will be weaker in comparison with the length of sleeping time if the time taken by stage 1 is longer.
- *Non-REM sleep stage 2 (simple memory storage)*: This is a stage of shallow sleep, accounting for 45% to 50% of the total sleeping time, which is indispensable for remembering the fractional pieces of information received in a day.
- *Non-REM sleep stage 3 (fatigue recovery)*: This stage is indispensable for fatigue recovery. Slow brain waves are generated in this stage of sleeping, which accounts for 13% to 23% of the entire sleeping time. In this stage, fatigued muscles are slowly relaxed; depleted energy is regenerated; and growth hormones, necessary for cell regeneration, are secreted. Fatigue will not be relieved irrespective of the length of sleeping time if stages 1 and 2 are repeated due to external stimuli, and it is for this reason that a long sound sleep is necessary without awakening, once a person has fallen asleep.

## 13.1   REM sleep (memory integration)

Why do aged people often not sleep for a long time? Diverse physiological changes occur due to aging. Sleep also changes with age and, as a result, instances of early evening sleep increase and instances of sleep at dawn decrease. The reason for this advancement of sleeping time is that the cycle of the living body clock, which adjusts the time for falling asleep, is shortened. Meanwhile, awakening at dawn and suffering from difficulties in falling asleep again will not be experienced if a long sleep is taken, even if the time for falling asleep has been advanced.

However, elderly people cannot sleep for a long time because although non-REM sleep and REM sleep are repeated in 90-minute cycles, non-REM sleep (deep sleep) decreases with age, while REM sleep increases with age. In childhood and adolescence, the ratio of slow-wave sleep (deep sleep in which growth hormone is secreted) is high. Elderly people, having shallow sleep, frequently awake to twist and turn and then eventually awake completely. Second, elderly people take many naps, whereas children aged less than five years old sleep twice a day. However, children who are becoming adults exhibit a long sleep only at night and, upon attaining an age older than 55 years, feel sleepy often and take naps even during the day. As a result, they cannot have a deep sleep at night.

Sleep is controlled by the brain. The sleep center is present in the brain and induces a person to fall asleep or stay awake. The cells constituting the sleep center get destroyed as a person grows older and, consequently, the signals that induce the person to fall asleep cannot be generated as strongly or continuously. Aging also reduces the secretion of melatonin, a sleep-inducing hormone. The quantity of melatonin in elderly persons is extremely low—less than one-fifth of that in children.

Various physical and mental diseases increase in people with old age. The most common cause of insomnia is pain associated with such conditions. Many elderly people have chronic diseases, such as arthritis, that are accompanied by pain. In addition, the use of various drugs (hypotensive drugs, anti-depressants) for hypertension, diabetes, and so on may also cause insomnia. Other diseases that increase with age include sleep apnea, which is the stoppage of breathing during sleep, thereby leading to shallow sleep, and restless legs syndrome, which causes difficulties in falling asleep with discomfort present in the lower limbs before falling asleep.

Mental problems such as depression and anxiety occurring due to emotional changes that present as people grow older are also important causes of sleep disorders. Elderly people should seek professional help if these problems persist, since sleep disorders of the elderly may be caused by physiological changes due to aging, medical diseases, and other disorders. Elderly people should practice normal sleeping habits, since they may experience chronic fatigue and forgetfulness if insomnia is neglected. An ideal sleeping time length for elderly people is seven hours and 30 minutes.

## 13.2    Symptoms of insomnia

A person will be diagnosed with insomnia if the symptoms that make falling asleep difficult, cause awakening from sleep early in the morning, and lead to difficulties in falling asleep again persist for at least one month, and cause problems in working during the daytime. The causes of insomnia are diverse, including psychological factors such as stress and worry, mental problems such as depression and anxiety, and sleep disorders such as restless legs syndrome (symptoms include discomfort in the legs prior to falling asleep). Sleep-related breathing disorders; various drugs (antihypertensive drugs, alcohol, adrenocortical hormone drugs, bronchodilators, analgesics, thyroid hormone drugs, opiates, analeptics, antidepressants with arousal actions); chronic diseases (arthritis, heart diseases, hypertension, menopause, pregnancy, asthma, gastroesophageal reflux, infection, stroke, convulsive diseases, Parkinson's disease, chronic respiratory diseases, and pain-inducing diseases); and poor sleep hygiene, including irregular sleep habits, can keep up insomnia.

Insomnia usually persists when it is not treated actively. Epidemiological studies have reported that insomnia persisted for at least one year in 80% of people having insomnia and for more than five years in at least 50% of people having insomnia, clearly indicating that insomnia becomes chronic in quite a few cases. Therefore, insomnia should be treated because it not only severely undermines daytime functions but also acts as a depression-inducing factor. Depression is said to occur in approximately 30% of insomnia patients. Insomnia and depression are closely related with each other, since approximately 90% of depression patients complain of insomnia. However, both insomnia and depression can be prevented through early treatment.

Insomnia degrades cognitive functions such as concentration and memory, leading to depression, anxiety, palpitations (excessive heart beats that can be felt by the patient), dysesthesia, daytime sleepiness, fatigue, and drowsiness. Insomnia also impairs concentration, causes memory loss, and increases the risk of accidents, while driving in a drowsy state. Insomnia symptoms not only cause learning disabilities but also severely degrade work efficiency. Social costs due to insomnia are estimated to be so large that their extent cannot be measured.

## 13.3   Sleep hygiene and nondrug treatment

Conditions helpful for sleep such as restrained drinking and smoking and exercising for sleep health in order to maintain health are referred to as *sleep hygiene*.

- The maintenance of a regular sleep-wake rhythm is most significantly emphasized for good sleep hygiene. Awaking from sleep at a certain time in the morning is important for maintaining this rhythm.
- Exposure to sunlight for 40 minutes to one hour, immediately after getting up early in the morning, is recommended because exposure to sunlight sends signals to the sleep-wake control center, indicating that daytime has begun while promoting the secretion of melatonin at night. During daytime, naps should not be taken for as long as possible and the time length of lying down should be reduced because a hormone that facilitates sound sleep at night is secreted during activities and sound sleep is possible only when an appropriate amount of this hormone accumulates.
- Taking a nap or lying down reduces secretion of this hormone so that the person in question must stay awake for late hours, in order for the hormone to reach appropriate amounts. Some studies have

indicated that the amount of melatonin secreted at night increased three to four times in people who were exposed to sunlight early in the morning in comparison with in people who were not exposed to sunlight, and this helped them to better fall asleep at night.

- Regular exercise helps in achieving a deep sleep. The time of exercise is also important. Exercising should be avoided immediately before going to bed because the performance of strenuous exercise before going to bed arouses the brain (including activation of the sympathetic nervous system) and body temperature, making it difficult to fall asleep.
- Coffee, smoking, and drinking should be avoided because coffee and smoking deactivate adenosine* (one of the hormones secreted in the human body that has the effect to facilitate sound sleep) and activate the brain, while drinking facilitates falling asleep through sedative effect but disturbs sleep by segmenting sleep.
- Abdominal respiration and meditation that relax the body and mind are helpful. Bathing in warm water is also helpful.
- Brightness should be appropriately adjusted since the presence of excessive bright lighting in the bedroom or living room in the evening suppresses the secretion of melatonin (whose presence facilitates falling asleep because it is a hormone secreted only in darkness) and disturbs sound sleep. Excess intake of water or food in the evening also leads to frequent awakening from sleep.
- If necessary, taking a nap for not more than 30 minutes is recommended because lying down for a long time or taking a long nap in the daytime disturbs night sleep.

Among sleep treatments, drug treatment is problematic because it has side effects such as a feeling of not being refreshed after sleeping, sleepiness, or a decline of cognitive functions in daytime, following drug intake. Recently, cognitive behavioral therapy for insomnia (also called nondrug treatment) has been widely implemented, mainly in the United States. A program aimed at altering various behavioral patterns that occur when insomnia patients try to sleep (because their anxiety associated with sleep is severe) is used in this treatment. Initially, during the education on sleep, in this treatment, the conditions that facilitate sound sleep are emphasized, rather than it attempting to control sleep through explanations about various factors affecting sleep and insomnia.

The most important concept is that out of 24 hours in a day, people should be sufficiently active for approximately 16 hours. During daytime, most insomnia patients lie down and try to sleep whenever they have

---

* *Adenosine*: A component of ribonucleic acid, adenosine triphosphate, nicotinamide adenine dinucleotide, and flavin adenine dinucleotide in the living body.

time because they cannot sleep at night. However, carrying out physical and mental activities during the daytime is rather helpful for night sleep. Although taking a nap for approximately 30 minutes is recommended, not taking any nap at all is helpful for sleep hygiene. Thereafter, in actuality, the necessary sleeping time should be determined through relaxation therapy, continuous checking of sleep hygiene, and a reduction of excessive time of lying down.

Some insomnia patients have distorted cognition about the disorder, for instance thinking that if they do not sleep for eight hours, that such may damage their health and they might die early as a result. Patients should be encouraged to move away from this notion by making efforts to change their distorted cognition by making them understand that maintaining health does not necessarily require eight hours of sleep per day.

## 13.4 Development of sleep inducers from shellfishes

A total of 10 kinds of shellfishes (*Mactra veneriformis* [MV], *Saxidomus purpurata* [SP], *Patinopecten yessoensis* [scallop; AN], gastropods [NC], short-neck clams [RV], *Atrina pectinata* [AP], *Meretrix lusoria* [MS], *Anadara granosa* [TG], *Cyclina sinensis* [CS], and mussels [ME]), extensively consumed in South Korea, were selected, and their sleep-inducing effects were compared in order to develop materials for sleep induction. Sleep-inducing effects were measured after oral administration of each of the 10 kinds of candidate materials to mice at a dose of 1,000 mg/kg body weight, and results showed that the ME extract decreased sleep latency while increasing sleep duration, thereby indicating that ME have the best sleep-inducing effect.

The sleep improvement effects of the commercially available sleeping pill diazepam and the ME extract were compared through pentobarbital* experiments. The results revealed that increasing concentrations of the ME extract decreased sleep latency, in that mice began to fall asleep, while sleep duration increased by 34% at the dose of 1,000 mg/kg body weight (Figure 13.1). Therefore, these results indicated that the ME extract had a sleep-inducing effect similar to that of diazepam.

The results obtained from sleep polysomnography,† as applied to human subjects, considering the results obtained from animal experiments, revealed that the wake after sleep onset (WASO), which is the sum of the increments in sleep duration in sleep stage 3, a measure of

---

\* *Pentobarbital*: A white, fine powder that is used as a sedative and a hypnotic. It is administered orally.
† *Polysomnography*: A medical examination that provides objective data for accurate diagnosis of sleep disorders and that assesses the extent of these disorders.

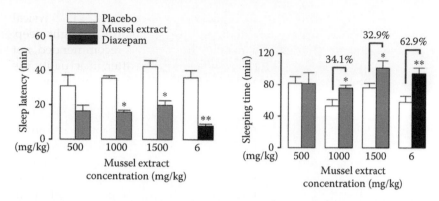

*Figure 13.1* Sleep-inducing effects of ME extract in an animal model (imprinting control region mice).

*Table 13.1* Sleep polysomnography of human subjects

| | Placebo | | ME extract | |
| Division | Before taking | After taking | Before taking | After taking |
| --- | --- | --- | --- | --- |
| Sleep stage 3 (%) | 2.3 ± 4.5 | 1.4 ± 2.8 | 2.4 ± 3.5 | 4.7 ± 3.6 |
| The sum of the time during which brain waves were aroused after falling asleep (i.e., WASO[a]) | 103.3 ± 59.6 | 61.8 ± 34.8 | 65.6 ± 79.7 | 67.0 ± 94.4 |

[a] WASO: Wake after sleep onset.

sound sleep, and the time during which brain waves were aroused, were improved, indicating the efficacy in sleep improvement (Table 13.1).

ME are shellfishes, and have a warm property that is good for managing weakness, increasing energy, controlling the viscera to enhance digestive functions, treating back problems and beriberi, and removing abdominal chill, in order to increase stamina. Among the shellfishes found in South Korea, ME are frequently used as food because they are produced in large quantities and their prices are low. In addition, they are not only closely related with the National Dietary Life but also regarded as sufficiently valuable as a new functional material because their sleep-inducing and sleep-improving effects were revealed for the first time in this study (Park et al., 2007).

*chapter fourteen*

# Antidiabetic effects of marine algae (Ecklonia cava) extracts

Diabetes has been known of for approximately 3,000 years and insulin, discovered by Banting and Best in 1921, represented a bright hope for its treatment. Diabetes will never amount to a dreadful condition if diagnosed earlier and appropriately managed, and patients who are affected can live out their allotted spans of life. No other disease like diabetes brings about so much happiness or misfortune, depending on whether patients have an accurate knowledge of the disease.

Diabetes is an abnormal metabolic state caused by the insufficient functioning of blood insulin. The most significant cause is heredity, followed by excessive intake of food, lack of exercise, and stress. However, diabetes can be prevented in a person who has a gene for diabetes through maintenance of a regular daily life. The onset of complications can be suppressed and a natural life span can be ensured by the introduction of an early treatment and care regimen, even when diabetes has occurred. However, a deep understanding and cooperation with the patient and his/her family are necessary in order to cure the disease completely. Although diabetes is certainly a disease that cannot be easily cured, the situation is not completely hopeless.

Diabetes is incorrectly recognized as a chronic disease that cannot be cured completely because it can easily recur if attention is not paid to the prescribed regimen, even when symptoms have disappeared and no glucose is detected in the urine. Therefore, a proper treatment should be given according to the physician's instructions and, if the prescribed regimen is continued, the patient can live almost the same life as healthy individuals.

The number of diabetes patients was not large in South Korea until the 1970s because the general dietary life was poor owing to socioeconomic backwardness. However, the number of diabetes patients began to increase since the beginning of the 1980s as dietary life became more lavish due to better income and improved standards of living.

## 14.1  Statistics of diabetes patients in South Korea

The recent increasing trend of diabetes has been occurring as a phenomenon not only in South Korea but also around the world. Some of the reasons for this include:

- The production of food in the world is increasing more so than ever before.
- The subjects under medical treatment are from developed countries with good food situations.
- Along with the development of medicine, the employment of early disease detection has also grown.
- The available treatment methods for diabetes have improved remarkably, thereby increasing the life span of diabetes patients.
- The populations at high risk of contracting diabetes have increased because the number of offspring of diabetes patients has increased following the extension of the life span of diabetes patients.

Thus, the lifestyle changes in modern people, including with respect to food situations, have had a direct effect on these increasing trends. The incidence of diabetes has been restricted predominantly to appearing in patients in their forties, fifties, and sixties, amounting to 70% of all diabetes patients in the last 30 years. The occurrence of diabetes in the majority of patients, after their middle age, is directly related to obesity.

Obesity is caused by the inability to balance calorie intake and energy consumption. Many people become obese nowadays due to a dearth of exercise versus energy intake, leading to many cases of diabetes. Although hyperglycemia is a disease that raises blood sugar levels, its resultant complications cause serious problems. Therefore, preventing and delaying the aggravation of acute and chronic complications by normalizing not only blood sugar levels but also hypertension and dyslipidemia are important in order to prevent the occurrence of vascular disorders.

Obtaining accurate knowledge on diabetes management and practicing the same with a goal of diabetes treatment should be a way of life. Above all, normal blood sugar levels (less than 100 mg/dL of fasting blood sugar and less than 140 mg/dL of blood sugar at two hours after a meal); normal blood pressure (less than 130/80 mmHg); and normal blood lipid concentrations (total cholesterol: less than 200 mg/dL, low density cholesterol: less than 100 mg/dL, high density cholesterol: at least 40 mg/dL in males and at least 50 mg/dL in females) should be maintained. Furthermore, weight control is indispensable not only for controlling blood lipid concentrations and blood pressure but also for preventing arteriosclerosis and controlling blood sugar levels. Diabetes, in many cases, is induced or aggravated by obesity and, in some cases, elevated blood sugar is controlled by controlling body weight only. Therefore, attention should be paid to body weight and a standard body weight should be maintained, if possible.

## 14.2 Balance between the size of meals and the amount of exercise

Diabetes treatment methods include exercise therapy. A person who measures his/her blood sugar level after walking for approximately one hour will find that his/her blood sugar level is below than that what it was one hour ago because exercise promoted the utilization of blood sugar. Hence, exercise is an indispensable method for diabetes treatment. Exercise therapy and dietary therapy for diabetes treatment can be said to be inside and outside together. Therefore, a person who considers their calorie intake per day as part of dietary therapy should also consider physical activities completed per day sufficiently.

Having sufficient physical activity is better in comparison with having meals that are low in calories. Depending on the size of a person's body, age, and progression of the disease, a doctor should be consulted in order to know how many calories should be taken in and how much physical activity should be performed. One can lose weight, be full of vitality, and have energy if the balance between meals and exercise is ideally achieved.

Proper meals and daily physical activities are the fundamental treatments for diabetes. In addition to meals and exercise, internal medicines or insulin injections are used only when needed. Diabetes is aggravated or relieved depending on the habits of everyday life. Type 1 diabetes is insulin-dependent, and occurs due to the insufficiency of insulin in the blood, whereas type 2 diabetes is insulin-independent, and occurs because the somatic cells cannot react normally to insulin in the blood and thus cannot absorb glucose from the blood. In both cases, cells cannot take up enough glucose from the blood, even if a sufficient amount of glucose exists in the blood. As a result, the cells, craving fuel to burn, use other body fuels such as fats and proteins. Meanwhile, the digestive system continuously absorbs glucose, leading to extremely high blood sugar levels.

Type 1 diabetes patients must intake regular insulin administrated through injections. Although insulin used to be extracted from livestock in the past, it is commercially produced these days, using bacteria that have been made to produce human insulin through genetic engineering methods.

Most researchers consider type 2 diabetes mellitus to be closely related with obesity, although this fact has not yet been elucidated clearly. Type 2 diabetes is controlled by regulating sugar intake, exercise, and dietary therapy for body weight reduction. Diabetes can be treated but not completely cured. Approximately, 350,000 people die every year from diabetes complications in the United States.

## 14.3    Antidiabetic effects of marine algae hydrolysate

The effects of marine algae extracts on the activity of the diabetes-related enzymes α-glucosidase[*] and α-amylase[†] were analyzed by Professor Jeon of Jeju National University, South Korea in order to verify antidiabetic effects. The enzymes α-glucosidase and α-amylase are involved in glucose production in the body by playing a part in decomposing ingested starch, and their functions are essential for maintaining the living body. However, suppressing the activity of these enzymes in diabetes patients is more important than anything else for controlling postprandial blood sugar levels. In fact, marine algae extracts have been shown to effectively inhibit the activity of the enzymes glucoamylase and amylase, and these results were similar to the effects of acarbose, a commercial antidiabetic agent (Figure 14.1).

Changes in blood sugar levels that occurred when marine algae extracts were administered to diabetes-induced rats and normal rats were measured, and the results showed a reduction in blood sugar levels in both the diabetes-induced rats and normal rats. In addition, marine

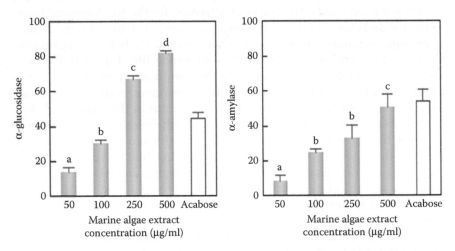

*Figure 14.1* Effects of sea trumpet extracts on the activity of the enzymes α-glucosidase and α-amylase in diabetic animal models.

---

[*] *Glucosidase*: An enzyme that catalyzes the hydrolysis of glycosidic bonds at the nonreducing termini of glycosides or oligosaccharides.
[†] *Amylase*: An enzyme that hydrolyzes starch, glycogen, and amylose.

algae extracts inhibited the formation of lipid peroxides, reactive oxygen species (ROS), and nitric oxide (NO), which were formed when protected cells were damaged by the treatment with fructose and the activity of antioxidant enzymes increased. Furthermore, marine algae extracts were found to inhibit postprandial increases in blood sugar levels in diabetic rats (Figure 14.1).

An indicator in marine algae extract that shows excellent antidiabetic effects was separated and identified to be dieckol. In order to experimentally verify the antidiabetic activity of dieckol, four-week-old rats were fed with general diet for two weeks and the antidiabetic activity was determined. Particularly, all experimental rats that ingested the marine algae extract containing dieckol showed a reduction in postprandial increases in blood sugar levels along with a significant reduction in fasting blood sugar levels. The marine algae extract group showed the stable maintenance of body weight and an improvement in blood sugar levels in comparison with the drug group, which showed side effects such as obesity (Figure 14.2).

Meanwhile, the antidiabetic effect of dieckol on congenital diabetes-induced rats was also verified. Dieckol reduced blood sugar levels quite significantly in congenital diabetes-induced rats (Figure 14.3). However, the efficacy of dieckol was somewhat lower than that of the commercial drug rosiglitazone, though it should be noted in this case that dieckol is not a drug but a functional food material. In particular, given the fact that the use of rosiglitazone as a hypoglycemic agent has been gradually declining due to several notable side effects (including heart disease and stroke), marine algae extracts containing dieckol are regarded as very useful substances with antidiabetic effects whose safety has been verified. In addition to reducing elevated blood sugar levels, the use of

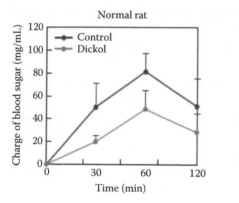 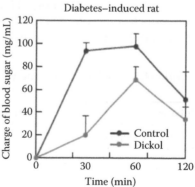

*Figure 14.2* Changes in blood sugar after intake of marine algae extract in normal mice and diabetic mice.

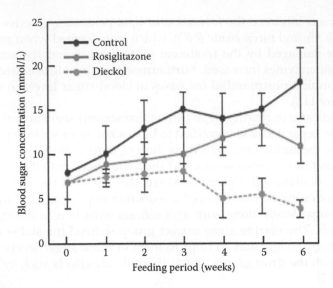

*Figure 14.3* Antidiabetic effects of marine algae extract on rats with congenital diabetes.

marine algae extracts showed significant reductions across all indicators such as plasma insulin content; triglyceride content, which is an important index of the neutral fat component; and total cholesterol content (Figure 14.3, Table 14.1).

Moreover, the significant decrease in glycated hemoglobin clearly indicated that blood sugar levels can be reduced by dieckol, as the decrease in glycated hemoglobin is not a temporary effect of blood sugar reduction but a result of blood sugar analysis that can be said to last an average of at least three months.

In addition, dieckol showed blood sugar-reducing effects in a clinical test conducted in potential diabetes patients using marine algae extracts (containing 5% dieckol as an indicator). The marine algae extract group

*Table 14.1* Results of blood analysis for antidiabetic effects of marine algae extract on rats with congenital diabetes

| Division | Control group | Rosiglitazone | Dieckol |
|---|---|---|---|
| Glycated hemoglobin (HbS1C, %) | 13.37 ± 2.72 | 5.43 ± 0.88 | 7.51 ± 0.38 |
| Plasma insulin concentration (ng/mL) | 0.64 ± 0.05 | 0.21 ± 0.02 | 0.29 ± 0.12 |
| Triglyceride (mmol/l) | 10.81 ± 1.41 | 7.78 ± 2.5 | 7.81 ± 1.97 |
| Total cholesterol (mmol/l) | 13.73 ± 1.27 | 7.56 ± 1.05 | 10.28 ± 2.09 |

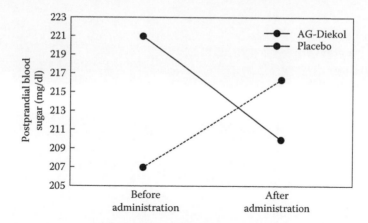

*Figure 14.4* Changes in postprandial blood sugar levels in a clinical test conducted in the subjects using marine algae extracts and measured 120 minutes after a meal. AG-Dieckol is the product presented in the marine algae extract.

*Table 14.2* Changes in postprandial blood sugar caused by marine algae extract use

|  | Before administration (mean ± SD) | Visit after the fourth administration (mean ± SD) | p-value |
|---|---|---|---|
| Dieckol (N = 36) | 221.5 ± 43.2 | 210.3 ± 46.1 | 0.0451 |
| Placebo (N = 37) | 207.2 ± 42.7 | 216.8 ± 48.2 | |

clearly showed postprandial blood sugar-reducing effects, whereas the placebo group showed increased postprandial blood sugar values, when the results of postprandial blood sugar measurements in the marine algae extract experimental group (indicated with the product name AG-Dieckol) and in the placebo group, 120 minutes after a meal at the second week after visit (before administration) and at the fourth week after visiting (after administration), respectively, were compared with each other (Figure 14.4, Table 14.2). This observation proved the fact that marine algae extracts suppressed the elevation of blood sugar levels in the clinical test conducted in humans, thereby suggesting that marine algae extracts, representing excellent natural materials, may be utilized as functional food and are also expected to help in the treatment of diabetes patients.

Measured at 120 minutes after a meal when the test subjects visited, dieckol is the product name of the marine algae extract used in the clinical test, and the placebo is the placebo group.

# chapter fifteen

# Allergy and marine algae

The Western lifestyle includes a healthy hygiene environment, which permits the occurrence of minimal infections; however, the changed physical state becomes vulnerable to allergic diseases. In addition, with increasing economic development, the rate of incidence of allergies has been enhanced, owing to the frequent exposure of people to harmful substances, such as air pollutants and yellow dust, and to indoor antigens and hazardous components that are discharged from building materials, forcing people to spend more time indoors.

In the 1990s, South Korea joined the ranks of advanced countries and, since then, the prevalence of allergic diseases, such as asthma, allergy, rhinitis, and atopic dermatitis, have rapidly increased by approximately three times; this clearly indicates that life habits and environmental factors significantly impact the development of allergic diseases.

At present, one in every three South Koreans suffers from an allergic disease, and one in five suffers from allergy-induced rhinitis and asthma. Recent surveys (Kondo, 2008) have shown that the socioeconomic losses due to allergies, including asthma, are considerably high. A study on asthma and allergic rhinitis was conducted in Asian countries (Shim et al., 2009), which reported that South Koreans are still not completely aware of asthma and allergic rhinitis and are unable to receive adequate treatment.

When the Austrian physician Clemens Freiherr von Pirquet first coined the term *allergy* in the early twentieth century, he referred to changes in the *way the human body reacts*. When an external substance enters the body, the body reacts in order to remove the former. For instance, when bacteria infect the body, the body generates immune responses to remove the pathogen, thereby protecting the body. However, if invasion by a foreign particle is tolerated in some regard by the body, the former may cause damage to the latter. For illustration, the unnecessary inflammatory responses, which occur when pollen is ingested, have deleterious effects on our bodies. Over time, the term *allergy* has been used to indicate disadvantageous reactions to harmless external substances, while the term *immunity* is known to represent beneficial reactions for the removal of harmful foreign agents.

Fundamentally, allergic reactions are physical reactions intended to remove external substances that have invaded the body. Therefore, in the context of the body, allergic reactions can be regarded as a part of the body's defense mechanism. Unlike immune responses, which occur in response to microbial infections, allergic reactions can occur as abnormal hypersensitive reactions triggered by harmless external substances such as food or pollen.

Upon invasion by an allergen (or antigen), antigen-presenting cells transmit signals to the type 1 and the type 2 T helper cells (Th cells), which trigger the generation of antibodies by B cells or assist in the activation of natural killer T cells (NKT cells), leading to the activation of β-cells (pancreatic islets of Langerhans cells that secrete insulin).

The activated β-cells release immunoglobulin (Ig) E antibodies, the binding of which on epsilon F receptors (FcεRI) on mast cell (connective tissue cells with unclear characteristics of physiological functions) surfaces activates the mast cells, leading to secretion of anti-allergic compounds such as histamine to trigger inflammatory responses. Therefore, the prevention of IgE antibodies binding to the FcεRI holds the key towards the inhibition of the onset of allergies (Figure 15.1).

Generally, allergic reactions are experienced in the body parts that are more frequently exposed to external substances. Therefore, airborne allergens that float in the air can enter into our body while we breathe, and can trigger allergic reactions in the nose, airway, and lungs, and may also cause eye infections. Allergens, if ingested as food or absorbed in the blood, are also capable of causing gastrointestinal tract allergies (leading to an

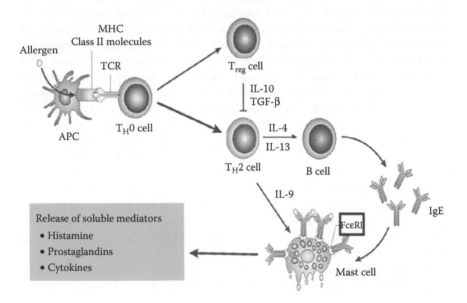

*Figure 15.1* The signaling system in allergic reactions.

abnormal increase in intestinal movements) or allergic reactions in the cardiovascular system and the central nervous system, respectively.

Once an allergic reaction occurs, immunocytes in the body that are exposed to that particular causative agent remember it, so that during a subsequent invasion by the same allergen, the immunocytes are able to react at once against it, resulting in either *dermatitis, rhinitis,* or *conjunctivitis,* depending upon the body part affected.

For example, the patients who are allergic to pollen show rhinitis symptoms, such as a runny nose, sneezing, and nasal congestion, between March and May, when the presence of pollen in the air is at its highest. These symptoms are generally silent during the other months of the year, but when the patients are exposed to pollen again, the memory immunocytes that were formed during the previous year's rhinitis episode get activated to generate diverse substances, inducing an allergic reaction again. An allergy continues to occur until the causative agent is completely removed or the inflammatory responses against the allergen are controlled.

## 15.1 Types of allergens

Allergens that enter into our bodies through respiratory organs are known either as *perennial antigens,* which can be encountered all the year round, and *seasonal antigens,* which are problematic only during certain times of the year. Typical perennial antigens include house dust, mites, indoor mold, cockroaches, and pet hair, while the seasonal allergens vary from trees in the spring, grass in the summer, weeds in the fall, and pollen that is extensively present in the air during other times. The most common causes of alimentary (food) allergy are milk, nuts, eggs, and soybeans in children and peanuts, nuts, fish, and shellfish in adults, respectively (Table 15.1).

*Table 15.1* Kinds of causative agents: antigens that cause allergy

| | |
|---|---|
| Inhalative | Pollen, dust, mite, dust fungi (molds), animal feces or dandruff, hair, cotton in furniture, spraying agents, smoke, and so on. |
| Alimentary | Eggs, milk, chocolate, fish, meats, tomatoes, strawberry, cheese, food additives, and so on. |
| Irritant | Gasoline, paints, chemicals, cigarette smoke, chemicals, cigarette smoke, cold air, irritant wastes, and so on. |
| Contact | Toxic ivy, dyes, metal materials, woolen cloth, cosmetics, insects, and so on. |
| Chemical | Drugs, diagnostic reagents, vaccines, insect stings, serum, Ig, blood, and so on. |
| Infectious | Bacteria, fungi, viruses, parasite infection, and so on. |
| Other | Physical overload, physiological tension, stress, and so on. |

## 15.2    Factors influencing allergic diseases

The rise in the incidence of allergic diseases is basically due to the inter-twined actions of genetic and environmental factors, indicating that the risk factors for the onset of allergies are more or less related with other factors. Hereinafter, the risk factors for the onset of allergies that induce bronchial asthma along with its prevention will be discussed in the following sections.

### 15.2.1    Antigen/allergen and prevention

Among the inhaled allergens that trigger asthma, the major indoor particles include animal-derived antigens, such as indoor ticks, cats, dogs, hamsters, and marmots and dust fungi, which include blue molds and *Aspergillus* species. Outdoor antigens causing asthma include pollen, dust fungi, insects, and cockroaches. In addition, some of the food components that may induce asthma include eggs, milk, flour, and buckwheat. Since these allergens constitute some of the major asthma-aggravating factors, appropriate management is required to decrease the proportion of such pollutants in the environment. For instance, as an attempt to improve the indoor environment, the removal of indoor dust mites (which are the most frequent allergens that trigger asthma) that may be present on the floor, sleeping gears, and granulated feces or insect pests, along with usage of clean duvet covers or bed sheets, is effective. The amount of allergen present in the environment is also related with the onset of asthma; it has been reported that up to 2 µg of the tick allergen (Der p) per 1 g of dust is tolerated by the body, but if the allergen's level exceeds 10 µg per 1 g of dust, then asthma is triggered.

### 15.2.2    Viral respiratory infection and prevention

Insufficient pulmonary function and accelerated airway responses were the symptoms that were reported in hospitalized elderly patients with viral respiratory infections. Furthermore, the morbidity rate of childhood bronchiolitis or the group morbidity rate was recorded as a predictor of acceleration of airway hyper-responsiveness, five years later. Thus, preventing the occurrence of such viral infections is an important measure in the prevention of asthma. In this view, influenza vaccines come to the rescue against influenza contractions and asthma onset and aggravation.

### 15.2.3    Outdoor air contamination and prevention

The potent mixture of nitrogen dioxide and sulfur dioxide at concentrations that can be reached in high traffic areas accelerates the airway reactivity of asthma patients to antigens. In addition, strong oxidizing pollutants such as ozone can increase permeability of the airway mucosa, increasing the effects of antigens. Towards this, the resolution of the global environmental problem will be an essential prevention initiative.

### 15.2.4   Indoor air contamination and prevention

Advancements in modern building technology have allowed for the prevention of outside polluted air from entering most buildings; however, on the other side, it has led to the generation of indoor pollutants, such as nitrogen oxides (including nitrogen dioxide), sulfurous acid, sulfur dioxide, and formaldehyde, from the heating of equipment and building materials and, due to the enclosed environment, it is impossible to avoid these pollutants. It has been reported that nitrogen dioxide, which possibly gets produced from heating apparatuses or cooking utensils, elevates hypersensitivity and responsiveness of the airways in asthma patients to even 0.6 ppm of allergens such as house dust mites. In order to avoid this, heating apparatus, for example, an oil stove, a fan heater, and so on, should not be installed indoors and rooms should be sufficiently ventilated so as to remove indoor pollutants that are generated from building materials in the rooms. As a precaution, care must also be taken to select new building materials.

### 15.2.5   Smoking and prevention

It has been revealed that tobacco smoke contains more than 4,500 types of compounds or pollutants. For the prevention of allergies, not only the asthmatic person but also the other family members must quit smoking. In the case of children, both the parents should quit smoking because the risk of onset of asthma increases due to smoking by the father of the child who has a disposition towards the allergy.

### 15.2.6   Food and food additive related prevention

The inclusion of food additives and Westernization of the dietary intake can be thought to affect the onset of asthma. Here, care must be taken to avoid the dietary components that are known to trigger asthma, or to refrain from the intake of highly pungent food items or the ones that contain sulfite. An improvement of dietary habits is considered to be an important factor in the prevention of asthma.

### 15.2.7   Exercise and prevention

The performance of exercise is one of the aggravating factors that causes short-term asthma attacks. Exercise-induced asthma can occur in any asthma patient and is attributed to a loss of heat or moisture due to excessive inhalation of air, which is colder than the airway and renders the latter dry. Likewise, excessive ventilation is also an aggravating factor for the allergic condition.

It is recommended for asthma patients to breathe through the nose and, if possible, wear masks. Prior to exercise, the inhalation of a β2 stimulant, aspirated suction of sodium cromoglycate, oral intake of leukotriene* receptor antagonist,[†] or continuous training for exercise may help to prevent the induction of asthma.

## 15.2.8 Alcohol and prevention

In the liver, ethanol is metabolized into acetaldehyde, which, in turn, is metabolized by aldehyde dehydrogenase (ALDH) into acetic acid and water. In the case of South Koreans, since approximately half of the ALDH genes are reportedly mutated, blood acetaldehyde concentrations are often high, leading to the release of histamine and thereby exacerbating the asthma symptoms. Thus, patients who experience alcohol-induced asthma are advised to stop the intake of alcoholic drinks or to receive asthma-preventive treatment after drinking.

## 15.2.9 Drugs and prevention

Aspirin or other nonsteroidal anti-inflammatory drugs (NSAIDs) are known inducers of asthma attacks at considerably high frequencies in asthmatic adults, but only rarely in asthmatic children.

Therefore, to prevent such problems, a prudent examination must be conducted to check if the adult patient has a history of an asthma attack due to aspirin or other nonsteroidal anti-inflammatory drug use; if found so, the prescription of these drugs should be avoided.

## 15.2.10 Violent expression of emotions or stress and prevention

Violent emotional expressions are increasingly contributing to the aggravation of asthmatic conditions by causing hyperventilation or hypocarbia, which results in the constriction of the airways.

As a preventive measure, both mental and physical treatments need to be implemented from the advent of asthma. In other cases, where an asthma

---

* *Beta-blocker (leukotriene)*: A linear chain of carboxylic acids with 20 carbons, which may block the beta receptors of endogenous catecholamines, a kind of physiologically active substance, to cause an asthma attack.
† *Antagonist*: A drug that plays the role of attenuating part or all of the action of another drug when used in combination with another drug.

attack is accompanied by anxiety and mood disorders, appropriate psychological therapy should be provided to relieve the psychosocial stress.

## 15.2.11 Other factors and prevention

Rhinitis, paranasal sinusitis, and nasal polyps (tissues that protrude with thin stalks on the surface of mucous membranes) can aggravate asthma, as these symptoms have been associated with asthma in several cases. Apart from the earlier, menstruation or overwork can also trigger asthma. Furthermore, complications such as rhinitis, paranasal sinusitis, and non-polyposis or gastroesophageal reflux require active treatment to prevent induction of an asthma attack.

### 15.2.11.1 Intestinal symbiotic bacteria and allergy

About 100 trillion symbiotic bacteria of at least 400 to 500 different species are known to reside in the gut of the average adult human. This figure of the microorganisms corresponds to 10 times that of the number of somatic cells that constitute an adult human's entire body. The concentration of bacteria varies in different parts of the gut; it can reach up to $10^3$ colony forming unit (CFU)/mL in the stomach or duodenum, $10^4$ to $10^7$ CFU/mL in the jejunum or ileum, and $10^{11}$ to $10^{12}$ CFU/mL in the colon.

Most of the intestinal symbiotic bacteria are anaerobes; some of the important ones include *Bacteroides, Bifidobacterium, Eubacterium, Fusobacterium, Clostridium,* and *Lactobacillus*. In addition, aerobic bacteria, which are present in very low amounts, include *Escherichia coli, Salmonella, Enterococcus, Staphylococcus,* and *Streptococcus*.

The gut of the prenatal fetus is aseptic, but after birth, microorganisms begin to settle in it. *E. coli* and *Streptococcus*, the aerobic bacteria, are the ones to occupy the site at first, followed by the growth of anaerobic bacteria *Bacteroides, Bifidobacterium,* and *Clostridium* after about a week after birth. The process of birth (natural or cesarean) and the status of breastfeeding of the newborn play critical roles in the settlement of intestinal bacteria. *Bifidobacteria* and *Lactobacillus* tend to be dominant bacteria in breastfed infants as compared with in powdered milk-fed newborns. Post-ablactation, the adult-type intestinal microbial flora start propagating, so that the entire gut microbiome gets gradually transformed into the adult type.

The established intestinal microbes, as such, are influenced by host physiology, such as pH and mucus composition in the gut, along with certain environmental factors such as diet and contiguous microbial factors like adhesion capability and metabolic ability. In addition, the interactions between microorganisms, such as metabolic antagonism* and the

---

\* *Metabolic antagonism*: Actions of substances that are metabolized in the living body and similar substances antagonizing each other on metabolizing enzymes, thereby obstructing the metabolism.

production of IgA antibodies and defensins (neutrophil antimicrobial peptides) are mediated by the host's immune responses.

External factors that immensely affect the intestinal microbial flora include antibiotics and meals. Recently, the role of intestinal symbiotic bacteria in the maintenance of the health of hosts has caught considerable attention. The intestinal symbiotic bacteria lead to the inhibition of the proliferation of pathogens and fermentation of undigested food.

The gut comprises the largest immune system in the human body and plays an indispensable role in the maintenance of our health. In addition to food, pathogens and viruses that are harmful to the body can enter the gut through the oral cavity. It is at this point at which the gut immune system accurately recognizes the intestinal symbiotic bacteria, food components, and pathogens, and specifically attacks the harmful agents for their removal from the body. In this way, the intestinal homeostasis is maintained; however, if at any time this balance is altered by factors, such as genetic background, environment, stress, or age, it results in the onset of conditions like allergies and infectious and inflammatory bowel diseases. Intestinal microflora is known to immensely contribute towards formation and maintenance of the gut immune system, as proved by certain experiments that were conducted using aseptic animals with no intestinal symbiotic bacteria.

In contrast with normal animals, aseptic ones demonstrate fewer elevated areas of lymphatic tissues in the mucosa of their small intestines, fewer IgE antibody producing cells, and fewer epithelial T-cells. A characteristic feature of such aseptic animals is the delayed immune responses following antigen challenges, such as the induction of oral immune tolerance.*

For normal maturation of the gut immune system, continuous stimulation from the symbiotic bacteria of the gut is necessary for the early stages of life. Oral administration of ovalbumin to aseptic mice leads to the production of Th2-type cytokines, thereby inducing the generation of antigen-specific IgE antibodies. However, the time of microbial stimulation is known to be important for the gut immune system: this is demonstrated by the fact that *bifidobacteria* induces development of oral immune tolerance only if introduced during the neonatal period, which its introduction at later stages is not effective. The immune system is greatly affected by microbial stimulation right after birth because it is during this period that the immune system accepts signals that induce its maturation when the gut immune system has not yet developed.

---

* *Immune tolerance*: Immune responses through which antigens capable of causing humoral or cell-mediated immunity become unable to specifically respond in lymphatic tissues.

The gut immune system regulates the health status of the entire body of the host. This implies that the effect of intestinal symbiotic bacteria is not limited to the gut immune system; indeed, the developmental abnormalities in intestinal microflora have been related to delayed maturation of the body's immunity, in particular, blood IgE- and IgM-secreting cells.

As such, the immune system of the host is delicately regulated by cross-talks with the symbiotic bacteria in the gut. Recently, allergic diseases, such as atopic eczema, food allergy, hay fever, and asthma, have increased worldwide and have specifically become a big social problem in the advanced countries. Since the genetic basis of such rapid changes could not be established, such a rise is attributed to the environment.

A 1989 study conducted by Strachan demonstrated that children who have many siblings are at lower risk of onset of allergy, as proved by the author's hygiene hypothesis, which states that the incidence of allergic diseases is inversely proportional to the number of infections encountered during childhood. Moreover, the survey results indicated that the occurrence of asthma is more frequent in urban areas than in rural areas, and that the rates of onset of allergies are low among children who started communal living at early ages (even before one year of age) in child-care institutions, and so on. The study also observed that children who are brought up in farms display low rates of allergy onset, further supporting the author's hygiene hypothesis. The hygiene hypothesis was first interpreted at an immunological level, in which it was found that the onset of allergy is suppressed because the microbial antigens induce transformation of Th2 immune responses into Th1 immune responses.

### 15.2.11.2 Inhibitory effects of Lactobacillus on allergy

In context to the relationship with microorganisms, the natural course of immunity development requires stimulation from bacterial infections. This is evident by the recent increase in the number of allergic patients in the advanced countries, where due to improved hygienic conditions, people are less exposed to infections and, thus, there is a delay in the formation of normal intestinal bacteria. Animal experiments have demonstrated that symbiotic bacteria in the gut contribute to the development of the immune system and that the host immune system is functionally affected by the former. Thereafter, epidemiological studies, such as one that compared intestinal microflora between allergic and non-allergic infants, showed that the number of CFU for *Bifidobacteria* or *Lactobacillus* spp. was low among the complete set of gut microflora of allergic infants or in the ones who contracted allergy at a later stage.

In 1999, Bjorksten et al. reported that the detection rates of *Lactobacillus* and *Bifidobacteria* were lower, while those of the aerobic bacteria (bacteria which require oxygen for their growth) were higher in the feces of allergic infants aged two years in comparison with those without any allergy.

In addition, the authors also reported that among the infants who were diagnosed as having allergic reactions at the age of two years, *Bifidobacterium* detection rates tended to be low until the infants attained one year of age. Such results indicate the possibility of the establishment of intestinal bacteria during the early developmental stages of infancy, possibly due to the consumption of breastfed milk that might affect the baby's immune system and subsequently trigger the onset of allergic diseases.

The possibility of *Lactobacilli*-mediated inhibition of allergy, which was demonstrated in a study conducted using experimental animals and cultured cells, was supported by the observation of the same effect in human clinical tests on atopic dermatitis (Kalliomäki et al., 2001).

With regard to the allergy preventive effects of *Lactobacillus* administration, Kalliomäki et al. (2003) reported that when *Lactobacillus* was administered to mothers before childbirth and also to the newborn infants, the onset frequency of atopic dermatitis decreased until the age of two years in the *Lactobacillus*-administered group. When the infants were tested at four years of age, however, the onset frequency of atopic dermatitis remained low.

*Lactobacillus* was chosen for such studies as this microorganism is one that actually remains in contact with the gut, which represents the largest immune organ in human body, owing to its unique characteristics of absorbing nutrition while being the forefront of the living body's defense against oral pathogens. The gut immune system induces unique immune responses, like the secretion of IgA antibodies and induction of oral immune tolerance, both of which are different from the immune responses triggered by other regions in the body.

IgA antibodies act on the gut mucosa to block invasion by pathogens, purify toxins, and stop the effects of foreign antigens. Oral immune tolerance refers to a phenomenon of the antigen-specific decline of immune responses that occurs when the relevant protein antigen has been orally administered in advance, in order to inhibit food allergies.

### 15.2.11.3   Atopy inhibitory effect of the dieckol separated from marine algae

Since a skin irritation may exacerbate atopic dermatitis, each factor should be well-understood for prevention of the allergic condition. In this respect, it was recently identified that *dieckol*, which is isolated from the extract of *Ecklonia cava* (a type of marine algae), is effective against atopy (an inflammatory skin disease). As a matter of fact, when an animal model (hair-removed), to which atopy was induced, was treated with a marine algae extract containing dieckol, not only was a reduction in dead skin cells but also remarkable hair growth observed (Figure 15.2). On the contrary, no such regain of hair was recorded in the non-treated atopy-induced animals, a finding which clearly indicated

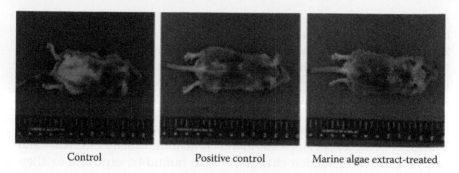

| Control | Positive control | Marine algae extract-treated |

*Figure 15.2* The inhibitory effects of marine algae extracts on induced atopy in an animal model.

that the administration of a marine algae extract containing dieckol is an excellent remedy for relief of atopy.

In addition, atopic diseases can be influenced by close interactions of immune system components. When IgE antibodies bind to FcεRI, which is a high-affinity IgE receptor, on the surface of mast cells, various chemical transmitters, including histamine, are released for immediate induction of allergy. Therefore, the inhibition of the high-affinity binding of the IgE antibody to the FcεRI receptor can prevent the onset of atopic diseases via the suppression of the secretion of anti-inflammatory compounds, such as histamine. Toward this end, we have demonstrated that dieckol extracted from marine algae inhibits the expression of the FcεRI receptor, obstructing the binding of IgE antibodies and ultimately discouraging the incidence of allergy (Figure 15.3).

Marine algae are classified as a healthy food. *The Wall Street Journal*, which is considered one of the foremost global economic magazines, featured an article on the significance of marine algae in South Korea. The in-depth analysis and publication of marine algae in a positive light by this United States newspaper deserves special mention, as marine algae are termed *seaweeds* in the West, although they are considered to be *sea vegetables* and are commonly eaten in South and East Asian nations like

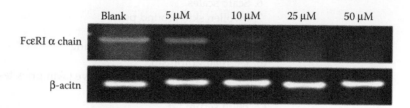

*Figure 15.3* The inhibition of expression of the high-affinity FcεRI gene by dieckol (isolated from marine algae).

India, Japan, and China. Among these, marine algae, which is a species of brown algae, has been reported to possess several advantages as a food item, such as that it is rich in calcium and antioxidants and is good for the skin, metabolism, diabetes, and hyperlipidemia. The fact that marine algae is beneficial in relieving inflammatory skin diseases and in improving atopy, was verified through the study conducted by Kim et al. (2013).

### 15.2.11.4  *Diagnosis and treatment of atopy*

The major symptom of atopic dermatitis is itching, which exacerbates and re-emerges due to sudden changes in skin humidity, exposure to allergens, irritants, excessive sweating, and mental stress. Due to unbearable itching, the patient feels compelled to scratch his/her skin, resulting in physical damage to it and further accelerating the inflammatory response. Such a situation leads to the continuation of a vicious cycle wherein repeated induction for itching gets maintained (Table 15.2).

The laboratory examination of an atopic dermatitis patient is not an absolute requirement for the diagnosis and treatment: however, it may help in determining the condition of the patient and the exacerbating factors.

*Table 15.2* South Korean atopic dermatitis diagnostic criteria

| | |
|---|---|
| Major findings | 1. Itching |
| | 2. Shapes and distribution of characteristic lesions |
| |    a. Infants aged less than two years: face, trunk, extension regions of the extremities |
| |    b. Infants aged two years or more: face, neck, flexion regions of the extremities |
| | 3. Medical history or family history of atopic disease (atopic dermatitis, asthma, allergic rhinitis) |
| Survey subject (name) | 1. Xeroderma |
| | 2. Pityriasis alba (ringworm) |
| | 3. Eyelid dermatitis and surrounding dark skin |
| | 4. Eczema around the ears |
| | 5. Non-specific dermatitis on the hands/feet |
| | 6. Scalp scales |
| | 7. Swollen skin around pores |
| | 8. Nipple eczema |
| | 9. Sweating accompanied by itching |
| | 10. Dermatographism |
| | 11. Immediate skin reaction positive (skin prick test positive) |
| | 12. High serum IgE |
| | 13. Susceptibility to skin infection |

*Source:*   Korean Society of Atopic Dermatitis (2005).

The examination includes an estimation of serum IgE and eosinophil levels, an analysis of the specificity of IgE antibodies to food, and the detection of inhaled antigens if any are present.

### 15.2.11.4.1 Atopy treatment

Treatment for atopic dermatitis includes a regimen of moisture maintenance of dry skin and the prescription of adrenocorticosteroids (for the treatment of dermatitis), immunomodulators, and anti-histamine agents (to relieve itching). The treatment guidelines for atopic dermatitis as set by the Korean Society of Atopic Dermatitis (KSAD) are classified into basic treatment; adjuvant treatment; and selective treatment, including maintenance therapies to prevent recurrence of the lesions (Figure 15.4).

However, since any kind of skin irritation can cause atopic dermatitis, all the possible exacerbating factors should be well understood for an efficient prevention of exacerbation of atopic dermatitis.

#### 15.2.11.4.1.1 Basic treatment

Basic treatment includes moisturizing the skin, the application of topical steroids and topical calcineurin inhibitors, and the removal of exacerbation factors.

1. *Moisturizing*:

    Moisturizing constitutes the most important basic treatment because damage to the innate skin barrier is an important etiology of atopic dermatitis and the skin barrier function keeps declining with increasing severity of atopic dermatitis.

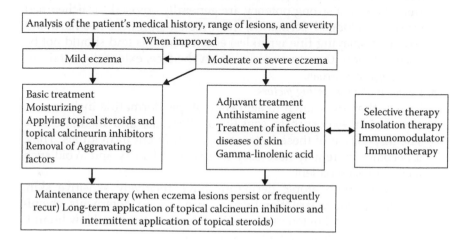

*Figure 15.4* Guidelines for the treatment of atopic dermatitis. (From *Skin Science*, Korean Dermatological Association. 2014. 6th ed. Seoul.)

The patient is recommended to provide sufficient moisture to the skin by bathing or taking a shower in lukewarm water for a maximum of 10 minutes, followed by an immediate application of a sufficient amount of suitable skin moisturizer on the entire body within three minutes of taking the bath, before the moisture dries out; this is recommended so that the moisture is maintained in the skin for a long time. Further, it is recommended to apply the moisturizer at least twice a day. The selection of moisturizer is based on the type of lesions present on and the overall skin condition of each patient, the season, and the patient's preference. Further, an oily cream or formulation can be used on areas of the body that are exposed while going outdoors during dry winters, whereas a moist lotion can be opted for use on the unexposed body parts, as well, during humid summers right before sleeping.

2. *Topical steroids and topical calcineurin inhibitor:*

Topical steroids are still considered to be the most basic and effective therapeutic agents for the treatment of atopic dermatitis, even though the controversy regarding their side effects has not ceased. These medicated formulations are capable of remarkably improving symptoms of acutely deteriorated lesions in a short period of time. Topical steroids are usually classified into seven types based on their strength, and their selection should be completed according the degree of eczema, the location of the lesion, the age of the patient, and so on, so as to minimize any side effects. Usually, the steroidal formulations are applied twice a day for the first week to relieve acute dermatitis and, upon marked improvement, the number of application or the strength of the medicine can be decreased. Topical steroids with a strong potency are generally advised for lichenified (during prolonged dermatitis, the affected skin becomes hard and coarse, displaying fine wrinkles) eczema lesions and should not be used for more than two weeks, or on the face, external genitals, or intertriginous areas.

3. *Removal of aggravating factors:*

Factors that are known to aggravate atopic dermatitis include skin stimulation, exposure to sensitized allergens, and mental stress. The disposition of these factors vary in different individuals. Thus, it becomes extremely necessary to actively identify and avoid such factors in each patient.

Patients with atopic dermatitis have relatively sensitive skin, which is prone to irritation by exposure to soap, detergents, chemicals, woolen and nylon products, high temperature, and low humidity, leading to the aggravation of eczema.

Various food items and inhaled allergens also cause aggravation of the allergy. Sensitization is identified by conducting skin prick tests or serological IgE estimation tests such as a mast allergy test. Food allergy is suspected in cases in which a pediatric patient presents with severe clinical symptoms and in cases in which symptoms immediately aggravate once the treatment is terminated. The major causes of food allergy include milk, egg white, peanuts, beans, and flour. However, unconditional avoidance of these foods regardless of the patients' conditions adversely affects their health and growth; therefore, it is important to avoid only those foods that have been confirmed to be inducers of the allergy by proper tests. Furthermore, such aggravating effects should be monitored periodically, as they are known to naturally disappear with age in many cases.

### 15.2.11.4.1.2 *Adjuvant treatment*

Adjunctive treatments include the use of anti-histamines, skin infectious disease treatment, and gamma-linolenic acid.

Anti-histamines alleviate the itching caused due to histamine release; however, since the latter is only one of the various mediators that cause skin itching, some patients do not show any improvement in response to anti-histamines.

Although hydroxyzine, a first-generation anti-histaminic with sedative effects, used to be the major drug recommended in the past, nowadays, second-generation anti-histaminics are commonly prescribed because of their anti-allergic effects.

Since patients with atopic dermatitis often present also with mycotic infections and may develop herpes eczema, in which infection by herpes simplex virus spreads widely, and infectious impetigo (inflammatory skin disease around the mouth and the nostrils), which is caused by staphylococci, relevant antiviral, antibiotic, and antifungal agents are advised to be appropriately and actively used.

Gamma-linolenic acid is an essential fatty acid component of the evening primrose oil and is known for its role in the treatment of atopic dermatitis by supplementing the essential fatty acid that gets reduced in the skin during the allergy. Moreover, the fatty acid can be safely used along with other treatments, as the former has no side effects.

### 15.2.11.4.1.3 *Selective treatment*

Selective treatments include light therapy, immunomodulators, and immunotherapy, all of which are used in patients with severe or refractory atopic dermatitis and who do not show improvement despite sufficient use of the basic and adjunctive treatments.

Some of the patients with atopic dermatitis who do not react to general treatments may benefit from ultraviolet therapy. Generally, ultraviolet A1 rays are known to be effective against severe acute lesions while ultraviolet A and B rays in combination with each other have been reported to be more effective on chronic lesions.

Immunomodulators include systemic steroids, oral cyclosporine, methotrexate (an anti-metabolite), azathioprine, and mycophenolate mofetil. Among these, cyclosporine is the most commonly used because of its relative safety and high effectiveness; nevertheless, periodic examinations are indispensable, as the drug is capable of inducing renal disorders and hypertension.

Immunotherapy involving the use of inhaled allergens has been proven to be effective against allergic rhinitis and in asthmatic patients and has recently been selectively tested in patients with refractory atopic dermatitis with positive results.

# chapter sixteen

# Effects of marine algae (Ecklonia cava) extract on asthma

## 16.1  Asthma symptoms

Asthma is a disease that leads to the narrowing of the airway due to allergic inflammatory responses, causing recurrent cough, dyspnea, a constricting sensation within the chest, and wheezing. Although asthma most frequently occurs in children, it also appears often in adults and the elderly.

Most of the patients with pediatric asthma and nearly half of adults with asthma have antibodies against allergens so that the asthma symptoms become more severe when a susceptible person is exposed to an allergen. Symptoms due to allergens present only in certain seasons or situations such as pollen appear intermittently, while symptoms due to indoor allergens such as dust mites and molds may appear persistently.

In untreated asthma, persistent chronic allergic airway inflammation leads to airway remodeling, and symptoms persist even in the absence of allergen exposure. Thus, early diagnosis of asthma and treatment of inflammation for the effective management of asthma are highly desirable.

The most common symptoms of asthma are shortness of breath, wheezing, and obstinate and persistent cough. Air enters our body through the nose or mouth when we breathe and it then travels through the airway to enter the lungs. The lungs deliver oxygen to our body and remove carbon dioxide from our body. However, patients with asthma have difficulties in breathing because the muscles that surround the airway become tightened, and the airway swells up due to inflammation and gets largely obstructed by the increased secretion of mucus. Therefore, when a patient with asthma breathes, a *wheezing* sound can typically be heard, caused by air squeezing out through the narrowed airway.

Asthma symptoms are worse at night as compared with during the daytime. The symptoms also become aggravated when the patient has caught a cold or has been exposed to irritants including dust, smoke, cold air, or pollens. The symptoms are sometimes aggravated when certain drugs or foods are consumed.

However, in fact, patients with asthma often complain of atypical symptoms such as dyspnea and dry cough without wheezing, and experience either pressure on the chest or a feeling as if the throat is obstructed by mucus, rather than the typical symptoms.

Asthma symptoms may be mild or severe depending on the degree of exposure to the allergens to which the person reacts; severe persistent symptoms can be fatal. In addition, the number of times of appearance of asthma symptoms may be different. The symptoms may occur once or twice per month in mild cases; however, symptoms may occur daily or throughout the day in severe persistent cases.

Patients with asthma generally show the aggravation of dyspnea in cold air and present with dyspnea and wheezing sounds most often during intense bouts of exercise including running. These individuals can catch a cold easily and, as a consequence, show common symptoms of cough and dyspnea for a long duration due to the aggravation of asthma. Therefore, many patients with asthma actually are not aware that they have contracted asthma and instead think that they have caught a common cold which has persisted for a long duration.

Since the causative antigens that cause asthma are highly variable among different individuals, patients with asthma should know the specific allergens that provoke their asthma and should reduce or avoid exposure to the causative allergens and irritants.

Once asthma has set in, the asthmatic patient is characterized by bronchial hyper-responsiveness. In these individuals, the airway narrows easily even with the presentation of mild stimuli, which are insignificant to normal persons. Asthma symptoms may be exacerbated by general stimuli regardless of the causative allergens. Representative exacerbating factors include exercise, the common cold, smoke, cigarette smoke, chemical substances, yellow dust, climate change, drugs (aspirin or analgesic anti-inflammatory drugs), food additives, and physical or mental stress. Becoming well-informed of and avoiding these aggravating factors is an important element of the control of asthma and the prevention of acute episodes A picture of *Ecklonia cava* is shown in Figure 16.1.

## 16.2    *Marine algae and asthma*

The chronic lung diseases such as chronic obstructive pulmonary diseases and bronchial asthma are caused by the complex interplay and interactions between inflammatory cells and cytokines (biological mediators involved in cell-to-cell interactions, including the expression and regulation of the immune response). In this context, macrophages, which are one of the cell types in charge of immunity, play important roles in the physiological process. When stimulated by harmful components and some oxidation products, macrophages secrete various cytokines (tumor necrosis factor-$\alpha$ and interleukin [IL]–8, IL–6, and IL–1) while migrating to the lung tissues. Consequently, those cytokines affect neutrophils

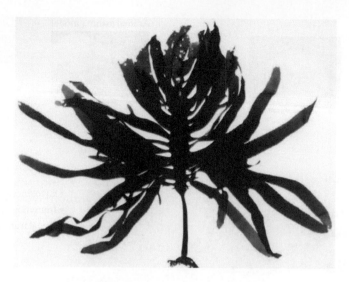

*Figure 16.1* A picture of *Ecklonia cava*.

(neutral white blood cells), T cells (cells that are involved in cell-mediated immunity while being in charge of the regulation such as suppression or augmentation of antibody production by B cells), and eosinophils (a sort of granulocyte among white blood cells) migrate to the lung tissues. These cells and inflammatory cytokines are important factors that cause chronic airway inflammation and remodeling. If these cells and the secretion of inflammatory cytokines are suppressed, airway remodeling can be reduced.

Therefore, as illustrated in Figure 16.2, an animal model was treated with ovalbumin to induce asthma, resulting in increased inflammation and secretion of mucosubstances in the lung tissues along with breathing difficulties. Subsequently, marine algae extract, which possesses various pharmacological activities, was administered to the animal model and the effects of the marine algae extract in the lung tissues were observed. Through the observation, as depicted in Figure 16.3, the inflammatory cells and mucosubstances (arrow) were significantly suppressed in the lung tissues treated with marine algae extract as compared with in the untreated asthma group.

Furthermore, the asthma inhibitory effects of marine algae extract were examined in cells from bronchoalveolar lavage fluid using a cell detection method that is used for the diagnosis of chronic lung diseases and respiratory diseases. The results demonstrated that administration of the marine algae extract significantly suppressed the infiltration of inflammatory cells into the bronchoalveolar area and decreased the numbers of macrophages and eosinophils in the marine algae extract treatment

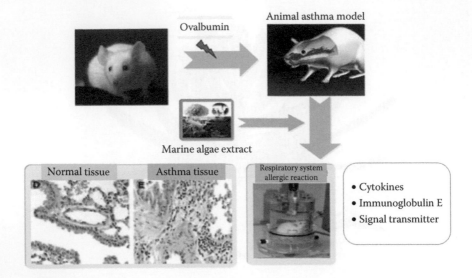

*Figure 16.2* An asthma-induced mouse model.

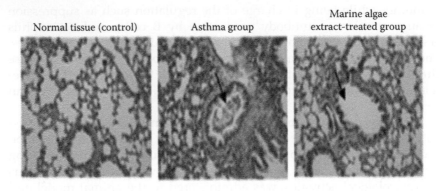

*Figure 16.3* Anti-asthma effect of marine algae extract in an asthma-induced mouse model.

group in comparison with in the untreated asthma group (Figure 16.4). Furthermore, bronchial responsiveness significantly decreased in the marine algae extract treatment group as compared with in the untreated asthma group in airway responsiveness tests (a bronchial provocation test) using methacholine. These findings indicate that coughing was relieved, which led to the stabilization of breathing (Figure 16.5). These results suggest that marine algae extract has potential as a functional anti-inflammatory agent for the treatment of chronic asthma diseases.

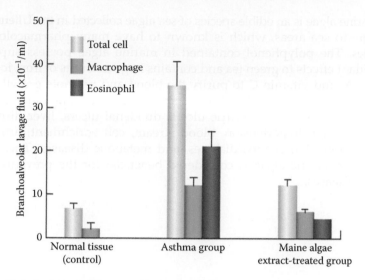

**Figure 16.4** Asthma inhibitory effects of marine algae extract in an animal model of asthma.

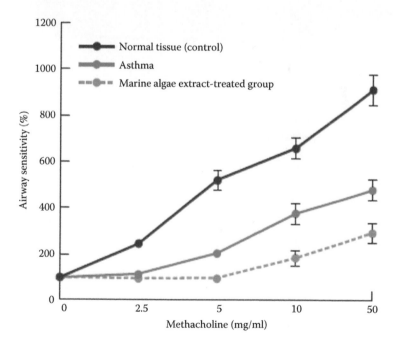

**Figure 16.5** The effects of marine algae extract on airway responsiveness in an animal model of asthma.

Marine algae is an edible species of sea algae collected in the Ulleungdo and Jeju-do sea areas, which is known to have many pharmacological activities. The polyphenol contained in marine algae possess superior antioxidant effects to green tea and contains large amounts of iron, iodine, vitamin A, and vitamin C to purify the blood and promote growth and development in children. In addition, studies have indicated that marine algae is effective against gastric ulcers, duodenal ulcers, liver diseases, hangover relief, hypertension, blood stream, cell enrichment, arthritis, inflammation, skin beauty, diabetes, and metabolic diseases. Therefore, consuming marine algae is considered beneficial for the prevention of various diseases.

## chapter seventeen

# Hair loss and marine algae

The Korean Hair Research Society has estimated that hair loss in South Korea affects more than 10 million individuals, and that 20% of these people are upset over their hair loss (Lim and Jegal, 2014). Consequently, various products claiming to be good for managing hair loss have been released. The market of options to prevent and care for hair loss— including shampoos and treatments, medicine and medical supplies, and wigs—has exceeded $922.5 million as of 2014 (Lim and Jegal, 2014). However, the ratio of medicine and medical supplies to other items in the hair-loss-related product market is insignificant.

In April 2014, *Houttuynia cordata* was made available in the medicinal market as a potential ingredient that is quite effective for hair growth (Figure 17.1). Shampoos to prevent hair loss became popular only starting in the late 2000s, and the number of shampoo items that have been approved by the Ministry of Food and Drug Safety only now reaches 323. More recently, observed responses to hair loss treatment devices that generate low power lasers have been astonishing.

*Houttuynia cordata* has long been used for the treatment of skin diseases such as athlete's foot and respiratory inflammation because of its strong antimicrobial and sterilizing effects. *Houttuynia cordata* was not originally used for the treatment of hair loss but has recently been gaining attention because it promotes hair growth and mitigates seborrheic dermatitis or seborrheic scalp inflammation. However, *Houttuynia cordata* is not considered very effective for other types of hair loss.

The beauty products including shampoos designed to prevent hair loss are divided into quasi-drugs and cosmetics. Quasi-drugs are those that have been stipulated by the Ministry of Food and Drug Safety for their effects to prevent hair loss and cosmetics are those that have been released without any particular stipulation. To obtain approval for the indication *quasi-drug* along with the indication *prevent hair loss and increase hair growth* on a shampoo from the Ministry of Food and Drug Safety, the particular shampoo is to be used by men and women (aged

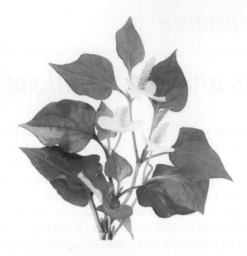

**Figure 17.1** A picture of *Houttuynia cordata*.

18–54 years old) with male-pattern alopecia for at least 16 weeks, the numbers and diameters of hair of the men and women must be measured, and the results should pass the relevant set criteria. Although shampoos to prevent hair loss may be more helpful in relieving scalp itching and in assisting with the removal of dead skin cells in comparison with general shampoos, researchers are skeptical about their effectiveness in preventing or treating hair loss because even if they contain good components to prevent hair loss, they cannot provide sufficient effects as they are only applied to the scalp for a limited period of time and then washed out immediately thereafter.

Low-power laser treatment devices to prevent hair loss show no thermogenic action while stimulating scalp cell tissues and promoting blood circulation to activate hair follicles, thereby providing auxiliary help for treatment of hair loss. In addition, low-power lasers have been verified for their effectiveness to cure wounds and to smoothen energy metabolism, and these effects are assumed to act positively on the scalp.

Terms such as *hair growth*, *hair-thickening*, and *hair-increasing* are being used increasingly ambiguously. When used commercially, these words may be misleading. The term *hair growth* should be indicated only in cases in which new hairs are reproduced at the same sites after hairs fall out, because hair follicles are not developed after birth in normal cases.

In cases where the hairs have become thin and weak due to male-pattern alopecia, the growth of thick and strong hair should not be referred to as hair growth but should be indicated instead as *hair-thickening*. This term should be indicated when the number of hairs is increased using artificial hairs.

Among the various hair diseases, alopecia especially brings about negative psychosocial influences on the affected individuals, although there are differences among different people. The numbers of persons who notice an unusually large amount of hair on the pillow when they wake up in the morning and those who observe clumps of hair falling out, resulting in totally smooth, round hairless patches on the scalp, are increasing gradually. Therefore, attention to hair loss, which was not previously recognized as a disease and thus was abandoned based on the belief that it was occurring simply due to aging or genetics, has been increasing day by day. Since the benefits of hair growth solutions claiming to be effective for hair growth in advertisements are not always accurate, the wig market has been growing rapidly in recent years.

## 17.1  Hair structure and functions

The hair follicle is a complex organ that is unique and owned only by mammals in the animal kingdom. Hairs are generally uniformly distributed across all of the skin, including long ones such as the hairs on the head, very short ones that can be hardly seen such as downy hairs, stiff ones, and curly ones.

Since human hair generally represents sex appeal and is part of body image, it is increasingly recognized as a socio-psychologically vital organ. Although hairs do not have any physiological function related to life as is seen with the heart or the lungs, the importance of hair is emphasized further these days as it affects every aspect of a person's life.

The head hairs provide protection to the scalp from sunlight, and the hairs comprising the eyebrows and eyelashes protect the eyes from sunlight, dirt, and sweat. The hairs in the nostrils and ears help to filter out the external irritants, and the hairs on the skin-folding regions function to reduce friction.

There are three types of hairs: lanugo hairs, vellus hairs, and terminal hairs. Lanugo hairs are very fine, soft, and light-colored hairs and are only found on the body of a fetus. In contrast, the hairs that remain on the human body during adulthood are vellus hairs, while the hairs on the scalp, eyebrows, mustache, armpits, and genitals correspond to terminal hairs. Terminal hairs are called as such because they are the last form of hairs made by the hair follicles. The vellus hairs and the terminal hairs are distinguished based on the diameters of the hairs rather than by the lengths of the hairs. The hairs that fall in between the two types, which are ambiguous to distinguish, are called intermediate hairs.

Human hairs are produced by hair follicles, which are a small but sophisticated organ (Figure 17.2). The epithelial tissues that constitute hair follicles originate in the epidermis of the skin. The hairs are produced

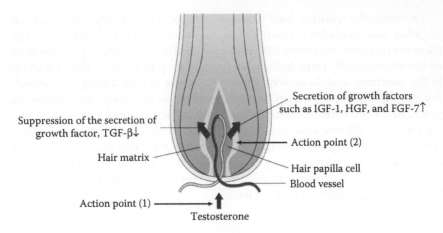

Suppression of the secretion of
growth factor, TGF-β↓

Secretion of growth factors
such as IGF-1, HGF, and FGF-7↑

Hair matrix

Action point (2)

Hair papilla cell

Blood vessel

Action point (1)

Testosterone

*Figure 17.2* Hair follicles.

TGF-β: Transforming growth factor beta
IGF-1: Insulin-like growth factor-1
HGF: Hepatocyte growth factor
FGF-7: Fibroblast growth factor-7

through changes in the skin. Between five and six million hair follicles are made in the cells during the fetal period.

In humans, hair follicle formation begins in the fourth fetal month of gestation, and no hair follicles are formed naturally after birth. Therefore, the number of hairs does not change throughout life.

A protein called keratin constitutes hairs. To be specific, the hair keratin is a tough protein related with hair. When hairs are formed, the hair keratin particles are tightly connected with each other to maintain the elasticity or flexibility.

To review the growth of hairs, the hairs of the fetus are called lanugo hairs and contain little pigment. Most of the lanugo hairs will be shed within the first month of birth.

Most of the head hairs in infancy grow up to 15 cm and turn into children's hairs. The fine, less-pigmented lanugo hairs that appear during the fetal life, and which convert to short vellus hairs during childhood, are called primary hairs and grow up to a length of 60 cm. At puberty, these same follicles begin to produce longer, thicker, and harder terminal hair shafts characteristic of the adult, and are called secondary hairs.

Both the hairs on the head and the hairs on areas such as the armpits, genitals, and male chin begin to become long and hard from the beginning of puberty.

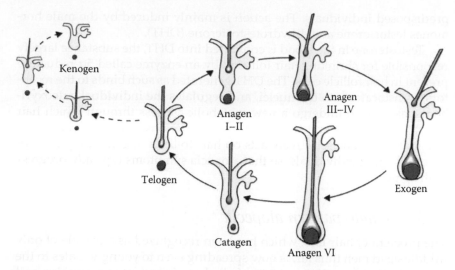

**Figure 17.3** Hair life cycle.

From the age of the late twenties, the hair anagen gradually shortens so that hair fibers become shorter and thinner. However, in genetically susceptible individuals, hard hairs are changed into soft hairs and the medical condition alopecia occurs.

Unlike other cells and tissues of the body, the hairs have unique biorhythms called hair cycles, in which hairs do not undergo the process of constantly growing followed by declining and eventually disappearing but instead grow constantly by approximately 0.45 mm per day during an anagen for two to six years, undergo a catagen for two to three weeks, and stop growing in a telogen for two to three months. On average, human beings lose between 50 and 100 scalp hairs on any particular day due to exogens, which is perfectly normal. At the end of the telogen phase, the hair follicles begin the anagen phase again and the cycle of hair growth continues (Figure 17.3).

## 17.2 Male alopecia

The bald head symptom, in which the forehead hairline gradually recedes or the terminal hairs on the crown of the head gradually transform into thin vellus hairs, is called androgenic alopecia or male-pattern alopecia. Male-pattern alopecia is by far the most common disease of hair loss. It is mainly caused by the action of the male hormone androgen in genetically predisposed individuals. The action is mainly induced by the male hormones testosterone and dihydrotestosterone (DHT).

Testosterone in the blood is converted into DHT, the substance largely responsible for shrinking hair follicles, by an enzyme called 5α-reductase present in hair follicle cells. The DHT generated as such binds to the receptors, translocates into the nuclei, and regulates the individual's deoxyribonucleic acid to undergo a new metabolic process through which hair follicles are shrunk and the growth cycle shortens, leading to baldness. The male hormone selectively acts on hair follicles in genetically susceptible and aging individuals, so that alopecia symptoms typically progress with aging.

## 17.3   Female-pattern alopecia

The problem of hair loss, which has been recognized as a trouble of only middle-aged men thus far, is now spreading even to young females to the extent that between 20% and 30% of all alopecia patients are females, and the number of females with hair loss in South Korea is rapidly increasing. Female hair loss can degrade the quality of life of patients much more so than in the case of a male with hair loss and is associated with low-esteem, a decline of self-confidence with respect to physical appearance, and psychological distress. Female-pattern alopecia is identified when androgenic hair loss has occurred in a female. Whereas hair loss progresses mainly from the forehead hairline in the case of male-pattern alopecia, hair loss progresses slowly during several years mainly in the form of thinning of the hairs on the center of the top of the head until all of the hairs in that area are lost in the case of female-pattern alopecia. The incidence of female-pattern alopecia is known to increase with age. Female-pattern alopecia is frequently observed in climacteric women, although it may begin in young women too.

A disease that can look similar to female-pattern alopecia is telogen alopecia, which is characterized by temporary hair loss due to the shedding of resting or telogen hairs. Telogen alopecia is a kind of alopecia that can be observed relatively frequently, and occurs because hairs in the anagen rapidly progress into telogen hair and shed before the end of the normal anagen. The most common causes of telogen alopecia include physical stress due to surgery; mental stress; endocrine diseases, such as thyroid disease; nutrient deficiency, such as iron deficiency; and drug use. The hairs begin to shed two to four months after the occurrence of one or more of the foregoing factors. Telogen alopecia is reversible, and hairs lost during this process are restored to their normal state over several months after removal of the causes. However, telogen alopecia may progress into chronic telogen alopecia, which persists chronically. Although female-pattern alopecia cannot be fundamentally prevented because it is hair loss due to a genetic factor, attention should be paid to prevention so that the rate of hair loss can be reduced.

## 17.4 Marine algae and hair growth

In South Korea, since self-treatment, which can be done in-house by patients, is preferred rather than medical treatment by physicians, unlike in other countries, the use of natural products of which the safety has been proved are typically adopted more frequently than that of commercial hair loss preventive products with side effects.

Therefore, to help prevent such alopecia, we have been studying functional materials for hair growth originating from diverse marine living organisms. Among them, the extract of *Eucheuma cottonii*, which is an Indonesian sea alga that has been known to be closely related to hair growth, was effective for the proliferation of the dermal papilla cells in human hair follicles and the root sheath cells external to the hair. When human scalp hair tissues were treated with the foregoing extract and cultured for six days, hair lengths were shown to have increased significantly by approximately 1.7 times (Figure 17.4).

Furthermore, when shaved areas of mice (C57BL/6) were treated with the marine algae extract, the telogen of the mouse skin tissues, in which no hair could grow, was transformed into the anagen so that the hairs grew; furthermore, the hair anagen-inducing effects were found to be similar to those of minoxidil, a hair loss treatment drug, as illustrated in Figure 17.5. The fact that the hydroxydihydrobovolide isolated from the marine algae extract increases insulin-like growth factor-1 (IGF-1; a growth factor consisting of polypeptides with a molecular weight of 7,500 structured similarly to insulin), which is a hair growth-promoting gene, was found, and the fact that the hepatocyte growth factor in the dermal papilla cells in human hair follicles to promote hair growth was also revealed, is important (Figure 17.6).

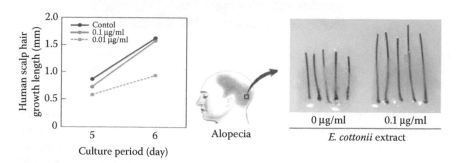

*Figure 17.4* Hair growth-promoting effects of marine algae extract.

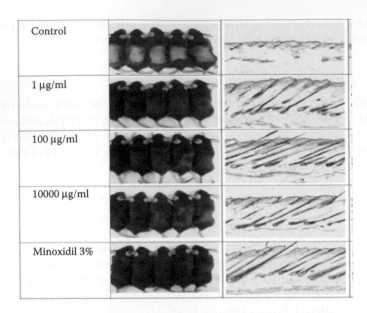

*Figure 17.5* Rat skin tissue anagen-inducing effects of marine algae extract treatment.

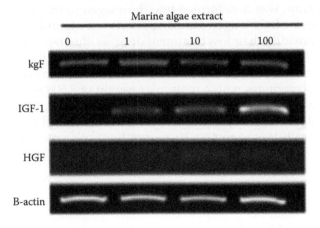

*Figure 17.6* Expression of hair growth-promoting genes induced by marine algae extract. Lanes: keratinocyte growth factor (kgF); insulin-like growth factor-1 (IGF-1); hepatocyte growth factor (HGF).

Based on the animal experimental results, a tonic containing 1% marine algae extract was prepared and a clinical test was conducted with the tonic. The results demonstrated that when the tonic was applied for 16 weeks, there was a significant increase in the density, thickness, and growth rate of hair, as shown in the photograph in Figure 17.7.

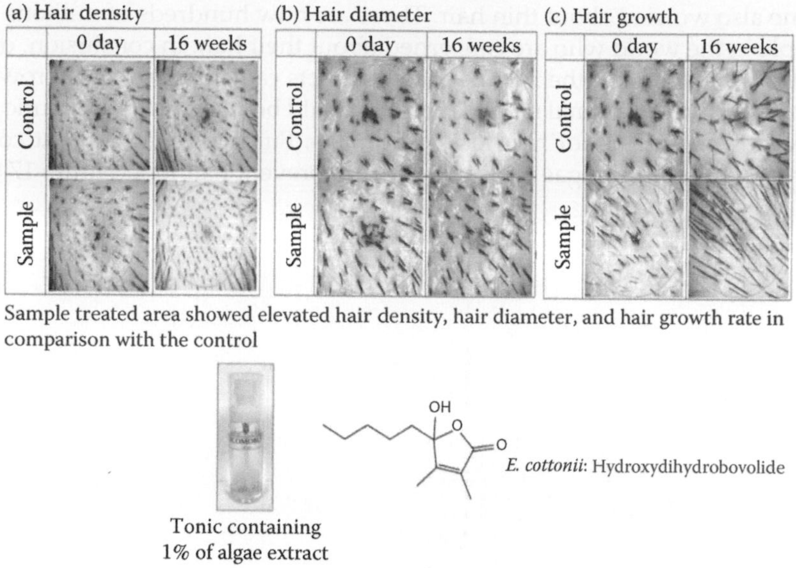

(a) Hair density          (b) Hair diameter          (c) Hair growth

| | 0 day | 16 weeks |
|---|---|---|
| Control | | |
| Sample | | |

| | 0 day | 16 weeks |
|---|---|---|
| Control | | |
| Sample | | |

| | 0 day | 16 weeks |
|---|---|---|
| Control | | |
| Sample | | |

Sample treated area showed elevated hair density, hair diameter, and hair growth rate in comparison with the control

*E. cottonii*: Hydroxydihydrobovolide

Tonic containing
1% of algae extract

*Figure 17.7* Evaluation of the clinical efficacy of marine algae extract for the prevention of hair loss and hair growth improvement. (a) Hair density; (b) hair diameter; and (c) hair growth rate.

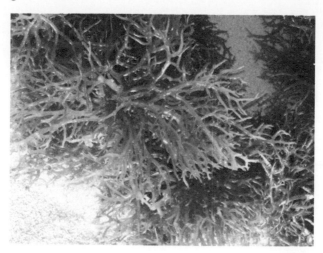

*Figure 17.8* A picture of *Eucheuma cottonii*.

The red alga *Eucheuma cottonii* (Figure 17.8) is marine algae which is mainly consumed in Southeast Asia, including Indonesia. This sea algae is rich in carrageenan and carotene and is widely used in perfume or hair conditioner. Aristotle wrote in the fourth century BC that it was remarkable that among all animals, only humans lose hair, and Julius Caesar in ancient

Rome also worried about thin hair. There are now hundreds of millions of people in the world who are concerned about their hair. In conclusion, our findings suggest that the marine algae extracts can stimulate hair growth significantly in an animal model and thus could be used as a therapeutic or preventive medicine for hair loss in humans. Furthermore, frequent consumption of marine algae is also thought to prevent hair loss (Figure 17.8).

*chapter eighteen*

# Acquired immune deficiency syndrome prevention by 6,6'-bieckol isolated from marine algae

In recent times, we have often seen or heard the word *virus* throughout social media. However, very few individuals know that diseases such as influenza that afflicts us in winter, the epidemic encephalitis that afflicts us in summer, and poliomyelitis that often affects children's limbs without mercy, are caused by viruses.

In general, much attention has been focused on viruses not only as pathogens that cause various diseases but also as important tools to pursue answers regarding the essence of life at the molecular level. Therefore, *viruses* can be safely regarded as living organisms into which great achievements of modern science have been integrated.

However, the existence of individuals apart from virologists who really understand *what a virus is* is extremely rare. In general, many people only have a vague understanding that viruses are a sort of infinitesimal microorganism and are pathogens that cause various diseases.

Although viruses are infinitesimal living things, they do not show any signs of life, irrespective of whether they are taken out of living bodies or put into test tubes containing an artificial culture medium. The aggregates of the particles are a chemical substance that is apparently not different from lumps of sugar. Although bacteria, which are low organisms, also breathe and ingest nutritive substances for reproduction, viruses neither breathe nor proliferate by themselves. However, once viruses have broken into living cells, they proliferate very quickly in large quantities. In other words, each virus particle has an amazing latent ability to replicate hundreds of identical particles. Once the virus particle, which looks similar to an inorganic substance, breaks inside a favorable cell, it immediately exerts its vitality to produce innumerable new identical virus particles in the cell at the rate of several particles in a minimum of 10 minutes to a maximum of several hours. Subsequently, these viruses become living organisms in the cells. However, once the progeny of viruses moves out of the cell, they become an inactive chemical substance, similarly to the parent virus. There is an air of mystery that surrounds viruses, which are like dormant chemical substances sometimes and living organisms at other times. Virus particles do not have respiratory and enzyme systems, which are considered indispensable to living organisms.

With this being the case, one important question is, then, *how do viruses proliferate?* It is a known fact that viruses can only proliferate inside living cells. However, the mechanism of proliferation of a virus is different from that of a common parasitic microorganism cell. Since they lack the substances and energy needed for proliferation, viruses borrow them from the host cells. Further studies are needed to elucidate the mechanism by which viruses proliferate.

Studies have shown that not only the filtrate (without bacteria) obtained by filtering the intestinal contents of patients with dysentery completely dissolve cultured dysentery bacillus but also the filtrate collected from the dissolved culture acts identically. This strange phenomenon, in which the effects gets passed on to subsequent generations, was first discovered by Derel in 1917.

Such phages and host bacteria are widely distributed in the natural world and are also found in the guts of humans and animals.

Phages can invade, proliferate, and destroy the host cells. Viruses that are parasitic on multi-cellular living organisms with complicated structures, such as animals and plants, infect many cells indiscriminately in tissues, thereby continuously proliferating in the cells.

Although viruses propagate at different rates, the number of times of a virus can proliferate can reach astronomical figures. Therefore, mutations allow for the occurrence of various variants. These variants or transformation of viruses are induced not only by mutation but also by genetic reunions, such as in the case of phages.

## 18.1   Influenza virus

Influenza viruses are ribonucleic acid (RNA) viruses that can be divided into three types, types A, B, and C, depending on their antigenicity (Table 18.1).

Although type A influenza viruses infect many animals such as humans, birds, pigs, and horses, types B and C influenza viruses infect only humans. In particular, type A and type B influenza viruses are seasonal influenza viruses that repeatedly prevail every winter.

In the case of type A influenza viruses, new viruses may appear to cause a pandemic because the antigen structures of hemagglutinin (one of the antigenic protuberances protruding on the surfaces of influenza viruses) and neuraminidase (plays an enzymatic role that degrades the

*Table 18.1* Forms and properties of influenza viruses

|  | Type A | Type B | Type C |
|---|---|---|---|
| Symptom | Typical | Typical (milder than type A) | Mild |
| Subtype | H1–H18 N1–N11 | None | None |
| Host | Human, birds, pigs, horses, and other animals | Human | Human |

glycoprotein membrane when virus particles leave the host cell) can easily cause discontinuous variations. The influenza pandemic has occurred at frequencies of once per 10 to 30 years until now, including four pandemics that occurred since the beginning of the twentieth century.

The Spanish influenza (A/H1N1) pandemic that occurred in 1918 led to the death of nearly 20 to 40 million people in the world. Additionally, the Asian influenza (A/H2N2) pandemic in 1957 and the Hong Kong flu (A/H3N2) pandemic in 1968, respectively, also led to the death of approximately between one and four million people. In the influenza pandemic (A/H1N1 pdm09) that occurred in 2009, approximately 15,000 to 20,000 people perished throughout the world. Although the mortality rate of this epidemic was smaller than that of the influenza pandemics that occurred in the twentieth century, it caused great social confusion, leading the World Health Organization (WHO) to raise the alert level to level 6.

The avian influenza virus (H5NI type), which is said to be the possible next new virus, presented in Hong Kong in 1997, resulting in the death of six out of every 18 infected persons. Thereafter, it occurred in China and Vietnam in 2003 and is now occurring not only in Asia but also in various other parts of the world. According to a WHO report, there were 668 confirmed cases and the mortality rate was high (approximately 60%) by October 2014. Human infection was caused by contact with infected poultry; however, the possibility of infection by contact between humans to cause a worldwide pandemic is still very low. In some cases, the mutation of the virus gene changes the virus to be more infectious to humans.

In 2015, the Middle East respiratory syndrome corona virus (MERS-CoV) prevailed in South Korea. This virus, which is known as the Middle East acute respiratory disease virus, is a new type of corona virus that causes a severe acute respiratory disease. Since April 2012, 1,154 individuals in 24 countries, primarily those in the Middle East, were definitively diagnosed with this virus and, as of May 21, 2015, 471 individuals have died due to this virus. Of all the affected patients, 97.6% were residents of the Middle Eastern countries such as Saudi Arabia and the United Arab Emirates; the fatality is approximately 40% and the latent period is estimated to be approximately two days to two weeks.

The Middle East respiratory syndrome corona virus (MERS) was brought into South Korea by a person who was infected with the virus in Saudi Arabia; it caused 186 confirmed cases and 36 individuals died, including those who were suffering from other serious diseases.

In the case of elderly individuals or those with an underlying disease, influenza is prone to cause pneumonia, which would typically become serious, through secondary infection by bacteria or mixed infection. The typical causative bacteria are *Diplococcus pneumoniae*, *Staphylococcus aureus*, and *Haemophilus influenza*.

## 18.2 The AIDS virus

The disease acquired immune deficiency syndrome (AIDS) was first known to the world in January 1981, when a 30-year-old male was brought into the emergency room of the hospital at the University of California, Los Angeles, United States. The throat of the male patient, who was identified as a homosexual, was almost completely blocked due to severe infection. Given that his entire body was covered by mold appearing like milk chunks, he had almost completely lost his immune function.

Although two more patients with similar symptoms subsequently came to the hospital and received treatment for several months, both of them subsequently succumbed to the disease. This disease was named as AIDS. The name means a disease in which the natural immune function is destroyed by acquired factors.

Human bodies spontaneously generate antibodies that resist against antigens that have infected them. These antibodies remain in the body for considerable periods of time, or even for life in some cases. They eradicate the same antigens that come into the body again. In addition, human bodies have an innate immune function that defeats quite a number of pathogens even without the presence of antibodies.

However, when the immune function has been lost, even trivial pathogens can cause fatal outcomes because the human body becomes completely defenseless. Therefore, it is difficult to treat patients with AIDS for even trivial diseases such as the common cold.

In addition, even if a patient with AIDS recovers miraculously, as may occur if the AIDS virus was found in the first stage, the patient eventually dies miserably due to secondary and tertiary infections. This is why the whole world is aghast with respect to the disease.

In the case of South Korea, according to the current status of AIDS-infected persons announced by the Ministry of Health and Welfare at the end of August 2015, the total number of AIDS-infected persons was 9,615 (730 females) from 1985 to 2014, and the number of deaths from 1995 to 2013 was 1,034 (Chang and Kim, 2001). Unlike other viruses, there are several stages in the diagnosis of patients infected with AIDS virus, as follows: (1) the latent period, a stage after infection but before the antibody is made; (2) the silent period, in which the antibody is present but no symptom is apparent; (3) the symptom period, in which the immune function has declined a little and various symptoms are apparent; and (4) the AIDS-onset period, in which the immune function declines very severely and diseases due to opportunistic infection that do not appear in healthy individuals or cancers occur and the destruction of the immune function by the AIDS virus cannot be prevented, even if antibodies are generated. Disease such as pneumonia, meningitis, and Kaposi's sarcoma appear in the AIDS-onset period.

AIDS infection is confirmed by serum tests after an antibody formation period for six to 14 weeks after infection and when the latent period ranging in length from three months to five years has passed. The initial symptoms (continuous dry coughs, diarrhea due to unknown causes, chills, fever, weight loss, and general fatigue) appear in 20% to 25% of infected persons, although the symptoms vary from individual to individual. Within seven to 10 years after infection, the infected person becomes an AIDS patient and the late period symptoms (swelling of the lymph nodes in the groin, neck, and armpit, and the appearance of purple spots) appear. Thereafter, the patients generally die within two years due to diseases such as pneumonia.

The WHO announced symptom criteria for the diagnosis of AIDS in March 1986, which are now used in various countries as grounds for the classification of patients.

The criteria indicate that there are three primary symptoms and six secondary symptoms in AIDS. The primary symptoms include weight losses >10%, chronic diarrhea that lasts for more than one month, and continuous or intermittent fever for more than a month.

The secondary symptoms are coughs that last for more than one month, itchy dermatitis, continuously occurring vesicular exanthema, mouth ulcer, esophagitis, chronically progressing herpes zoster, persistent esophagus, mouth and esophagus salt, and systemic swelling.

The WHO recommends the diagnosis of AIDS when two or more primary symptoms and one or more secondary symptoms appear.

## 18.3   What is immunity?

The AIDS virus destroys the immune system. This is the essence of AIDS. The various symptoms of AIDS are ancillary phenomena caused by immunity degradation.

However, *how does the immune system work?* Our body is an assembly of individual cells; there are approximately 60 trillion cells in the typical human body. When we think about the body, we usually do not think at the cellular level but do often think at the organ level, for example that the stomach condition is bad or the heartbeat is poor.

However, the poor condition of an organ should be considered as indicative of the poor condition of the cells that constitute the organ. For instance, the decline of the digestive function of the stomach indicates that the cells that secrete digestive fluids, such as hydrochloric acid and pepsin, have declined; the palpitating of the heart indicates that sufficient nutrients were not supplied to those cells that constitute the heart muscles, leading to the lack of oxygen, and thereby, making the movements slow.

Cells differentiate and form various tissues that play different roles. Among them, so-called army tissues that help get rid of invaders from the outside are known as *immunocytes*. Many immunocytes gathered together form the immune system.

These immunocytes attack any cells, viruses, protozoa, and molds invading from the outside and defend other cells against attacks by these invaders. However, some of the invaders break through the defenses of this immune system and become parasitic to body cells and tissues. Many invaders such as helper virus, hepatitis B virus, and carinii protozoa are parasitic on our bodies.

In most cases, their proliferation is generally adequately inhibited by immunocytes. However, the AIDS virus destroys T cells in the immunocytes and reduces immunity, thereby completely breaking the balance.

Although numerous immunocytes are known, three of them can be said to be the major ones; these are macrophages, T cells, and B cells. T cells are the central being of the immune system and are the largest in number and with diverse functions. There are three types of T cells: helper T cells, suppressor T cells, and killer T cells. Among these, the helper T cells and suppressor T cells function as a team and have completely opposite activities. Helper T cells activate B cells to make more antibodies. Conversely, suppressor T cells suppress B cells.

The immunocytes collectively attack outside invaders, and macrophages play an important role in the forefront during an attack.

Macrophages are cells in the form of amoebas that move in the blood by changing their shapes; they live in all tissues of the body. When bacteria or viruses have invaded the body, first, the helper T cells detect them and signal macrophages to approach the invaded region. The macrophages surround the invaders with their own cell membranes, confine them, and decompose and kill them with chemical substances. Macrophages release a substance called interleukin, which transmits signals between immunocytes. Interleukin-I activates T cells and increases their number;

the activated T cells release a substance called interleukin-II (IL-II), which activates helper T cells, thereby activating B cells.

Subsequently, the B cells begin to produce antibodies, which separate from the B cells, rush towards the antigens, and adhere to the antigens to destroy them. However, in cases in which bacteria or viruses invade when nutrition conditions are poor or fatigue has been accumulated, these immune cells cannot properly eradicate antigens. The antigens produced by B cells invade deep into the body to attack/destroy various cells, leading to diseases. In general, the disease is cured over some period of time as immunocytes move more actively. For example, when a person has contracted a common cold, the person recovers in two to three days if he/she intakes sufficient nutrition and rests; in these individuals, the immunocytes actively eradicate common cold viruses (Figure 18.1).

The AIDS virus invades into T cells, particularly into helper T cells, and proliferates while attacking the cells from both the inside and outside angles. It then repeats the foregoing process to keep destroying helper T cells.

In the absence of helper T cell signals, the macrophages, B cells, killer T cells, and helper T cells cannot sufficiently exert their abilities.

Therefore, *Candida* (yeasts that form cream-colored colonies by proliferating in the state of molecules without forming spores) or *Pneumocystis carinii* (protozoa causing pneumonia) keep proliferating and invading internal organs such as the lungs, digestive organs, and skin, eventually leading to death.

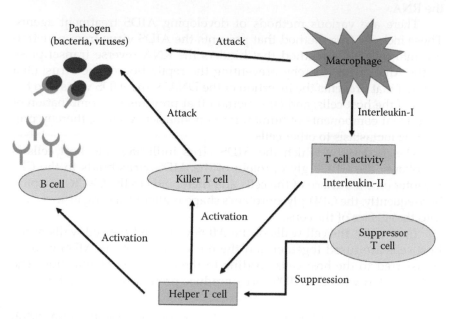

*Figure 18.1* The immune system.

## 18.4    *The AIDS virus that scatters the immune system*

In viruses, genes are packed at the center inside a protein coat. Unlike bacteria, viruses cannot proliferate by themselves. They enter cells such as animal cells and proliferate. When viruses adhere to animal cells or bacteria, they inject their genes into the cells or bacteria. Thereafter, they keep propagating their genes using substances or energy in the cells; these cells infected by viruses produce virus genes, which are surrounded by protein membranes of the cell. When viruses propagate extensively, they act on the cell membranes and rupture them; this is how they are released outside. Consequently, the viruses destroy animal cells and cause diseases in humans.

Similar to other retroviruses, the AIDS virus contains RNA as genetic material. They make humans more susceptible to other deadly diseases with their proliferation process.

Retroviruses have several genes that make proteins. Reverse transcriptase* is one of the proteins made by these genes; it is an enzyme that synthesizes deoxyribonucleic acids (DNAs) with complementary nucleotide sequences using single-stranded RNA as a template.

To prevent AIDS, it is essential to prevent the virus from entering the cells. Even when it has entered the cells, it cannot proliferate if the reverse transcriptase made by it is hindered because DNAs cannot be made from the RNA.

There are various methods of developing AIDS treatment agents. These include: (1) a method that prevents the AIDS virus from penetrating into cells; (2) a method that hinders the RNA reverse transcriptase of the AIDS virus, thereby preventing the replication of the virus; (3) a method that prevents the insertion of the DNA of the AIDS virus into the DNA of the host cells; and (4) a method that prevents the combination of individual components of human immunodeficiency virus, thereby preventing metastasis to other cells.

The process by which the AIDS virus infiltrates into host cells is as follows: the GP120 glycoprotein of the AIDS virus binds to the $CD_4$ receptor on the surface of the cells and then binds to the $CXCR_4$ receptor. Subsequently, the GP41 glycoprotein's shape is altered, aiding its insertion into the surface of the cells.

Eventually, the cell walls of the AIDS virus and the cell walls of the host cells are fused together and the nucleocapsid of the AIDS virus is transferred to the host cells, leading to the beginning of infection. The cells infected with the AIDS virus produce proteins necessary for virus

---

* Reverse transcriptase (RT) is an enzyme used to generate complementary DNA (cDNA) from an RNA template in a process called reverse transcription.

proliferation; these proteins migrate to the cell surface and then fuse with uninfected cells using the $CD_4$ cell surface receptor to form syncytia, which are giant fused bodies of cells. Syncytia formation is an important phenomenon in AIDS virus infection; the proliferation of the AIDS virus can be inhibited by inhibiting syncytia formation.

## 18.5 AIDS prevention by 6,6'-bieckol in marine algae extract

Utilizing this mechanism, we conducted a study in an attempt to develop a new AIDS treatment agent from the marine living organism. We concluded that when T lymphocytes (C8166 cells) were infected with the AIDS virus, syncytia were formed, but when the cells were treated with 6,6'-bieckol separated from marine algae extract, the formation of syncytia was remarkably suppressed.

In addition, to confirm the AIDS virus proliferation inhibitory effect, cells (C8166 cells) not infected with the AIDS virus and cells infected with the AIDS virus were simultaneously cultured and treated with 6,6'-bieckol at various concentrations. The formation of syncytia was remarkably suppressed in a concentration-dependent manner (Figures 18.2 and 18.3).

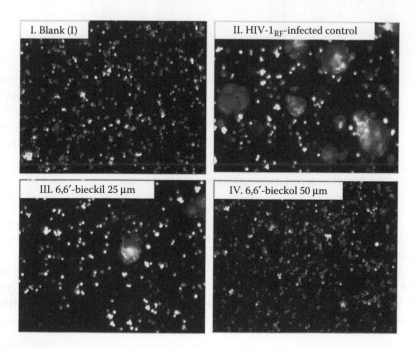

*Figure 18.2* Syncytia formation inhibitory effect of 6,6'-bieckol in C8166 cells infected with the AIDS virus.

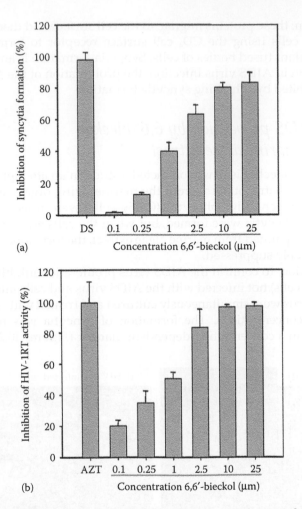

(a)

(b)

*Figure 18.3* (a) Syncytia formation and (b) reverse transcriptase inhibitor effects of 6,6′-bieckol in C81G6 cells infected with the AIDS virus.

In addition, the activity of reverse transcriptase, which makes DNA from AIDS virus RNA, was remarkably inhibited.

Therefore, 6,6′-bieckol separated from marine algae extract can be used as an AIDS treatment agent because it inhibits not only the formation of syncytia appearing due to the infection with AIDS virus but also the activity of reverse transcriptase.

# chapter nineteen

# Fisheries products and hypertension

In the age of modernization, *hypertension* is a term known to every individual. It is emerging as one of the major diseases, consequently resulting in a huge number of deaths worldwide. However, people with sufficient knowledge about the disease are not especially numerous. One of the primary problems associated with hypertension is that it causes serious complications. However, individuals with high blood pressure who are suffering from hypertension may neglect treatment because of their limited knowledge about the serious consequences of hypertension. The repercussions of noncompliance with treatment are not realized until they are encountered. Therefore, hypertension is sometimes called *the silent killer.*

To know whether an individual suffers from hypertension, an examination of normal blood pressure is necessary. The human heart efficiently and continuously contracts and dilates to supply blood rich in oxygen and nutrients to the entire body. Every time the heart contracts, oxygenated blood is spurted into the arteries, consequently increasing the pressure of blood in the arteries. Contrary to this, during dilatation, the blood pressure in the arteries drops.

The pressure in the arteries is proportional to the amount of blood pumped every time the heart contracts. The blood pressure of the body, in turn, is determined by the resistance provided by the arteries that obstruct the flow of blood through the blood vessels. The normal blood pressure of an adult individual is approximately 120 mmHg (known as systolic blood pressure) when the heart contracts, whereas the diastolic blood pressure is approximately 80 mmHg when the heart dilates. If the systolic and diastolic blood pressures are above 140 and 90 mmHg, respectively, then the patient can be defined as having hypertension.

Although no other disease is known as widely as hypertension, its cause remains elusive. Thus, many researchers are still asking the question, *why does hypertension occur?* For instance, a normal assumption would be that blood pressure should be high when the resistance of blood vessels is high, leading to a more efficient pumping of blood by heart to constantly maintain the flow of blood to the entire body. Then, one may ask, under what circumstances does the resistance of the blood vessels increase?

One of the primary causes of increase in the resistance of the blood vessels is arteriosclerosis, a condition manifested by the thickening and loss of elasticity of blood vessels, thereby restricting the flow of blood. In addition, blood pressure increases in certain situations, such as renal and adrenal diseases, and when oral contraceptives are taken. Such cases are medically referred to as secondary hypertension. However, in most cases, the exact cause of hypertension is unknown, and is thus a condition termed as *essential hypertension.*

Although the root cause of hypertension is not accurately known, the risk factors that contribute to elevating the blood pressure are well-known. Representative examples are genetic predisposition; sex, especially male; age; obesity; personality; mental stress; salt intake; smoking; and drinking.

## 19.1   Complications of hypertension

The risk of complications increases in all forms of hypertension, regardless of severity. It has been observed that the higher the blood pressure, the higher the risk. Another important thing is the concept of *high normal blood pressure,* which refers to a blood pressure value that is relatively high but that falls in the normal range. This condition is manifested by a high risk of future onset of hypertension. Moreover, the risk of occurrence of cardiovascular system diseases in these individuals is higher compared with in those with low blood pressure. The symptoms of complications due to hypertension are depicted in Table 19.1.

Most patients are insensitive to risk factors responsible for the rise in blood pressure, whereas hypertension is treatable if the patients stick to drug treatment. However, it should be noted that the hypertension treatment effect of anti-hypertensive drugs is temporary such that the blood pressure again increases when the drug treatment is withdrawn. With incorrect treatment methodology, even patients who generally begin the drug treatment in combination with other treatments refuse the use of anti-hypertensive drugs later, claiming the belief that once they have used anti-hypertensive drugs, that they should take them for life.

All of these may be attributed to a failure to recognize the importance of changes in the lifestyle that are necessary to remove the risk factors contributing to hypertension. Moreover, in the case of hypertension with mild symptoms, making a change in lifestyle habits to avoid risk factors are sufficient for treatment. These include changes in dietary habits, exercise, stress relief, drinking habits, and cessation of smoking.

*Table 19.1* Complications that accompany hypertension and their symptoms

| Complications | Symptoms |
|---|---|
| Atherosclerosis | Atherosclerosis refers to the accumulation of fat in damaged blood vessels, similar to rusted pipes. Although atherosclerosis cases generally increase with increasing age, this process tends to be further promoted in hypertension patients. Eventually, stroke or heart attack occurs. |
| Renal disorder | In the case of patients with hypertension, the arteries in the kidneys become thinner and narrower. Eventually, the ability to filter waste from the kidney is reduced. |
| Cardiomegaly | Hypertension compels the heart to work harder to pump blood. This leads to an abnormal enlargement of heart muscles, a condition not suitable for the efficient functioning of the heart. |
| Stroke | A stroke generally occurs owing to the blockage of cerebral blood vessels by cholesterol clots, which in turn, may lead to bursting of cerebral blood vessels. Stroke is fatal depending on cases or causes, such as quadriplegia and speech disorders. |
| Eye disorder | In the case of hypertension patients, small bleeding may occur in the retina that plays the role of sensing light from the inside of the eye. |

## 19.2   Table salt and hypertension

Essential hypertension is the most common chronic disease and serves as a risk factor for cardiovascular diseases, stroke, and renal failure. To study the relationship between hypertension and table salt, Dahl, in 1954, used rats susceptible to table salt as hypertension model animals to reveal the fact that sodium is a potent factor for the elevation of blood pressure. In epidemiologic studies, the effects of low sodium intake to lower the blood pressure and reduce the risk of hypertension have been recognized.

However, Whitescarver et al. (1984) suggested that anions, which are counterparts of sodium, were closely related with the elevation of blood pressure. Kurtz et al. (1987) reported that when sodium citrate that did not contain chlorine was administered to patients with hypertension with a mean maximum blood pressure of 159 mmHg instead of table salt, that their blood pressure dropped to 135 mmHg similarly to in cases in which salt intake was reduced but did not show the action mechanism. This observation forces one to ask whether sodium and chlorine in table salt are indeed involved in the elevation of blood pressure.

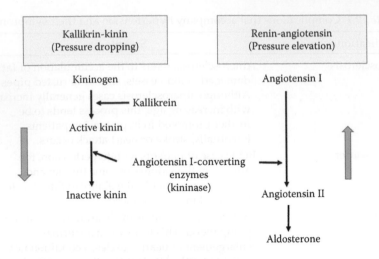

*Figure 19.1* Blood pressure control mechanism.

Angiotensin-converting enzyme (ACE) is a highly specific protease that plays an important role in controlling blood pressure and the body fluid volume. Angiotensin I is produced from the cleavage of angiotensinogen by the enzyme renin,* which is secreted in the kidney.

ACE functions by releasing two amino acids from angiotensin I, thereby converting it into potent angiotensin II, a molecule responsible for raising blood pressure. Therefore, ACE inhibitors are utilized as treatment agents for hypertension. ACE is present in the lungs, blood vessel walls, brain, and kidneys (Figure 19.1).

Kato et al. (2001) demonstrated that ACE, which plays a pivotal role in the control of blood pressure, is activated by chlorine ions in table salt. They found that ACE could be activated by sodium chloride or potassium chloride that do not contain any sodium, within the range of physiological concentrations. This effect hardly changed when added with sodium acetate without chlorine (Figure 19.2). Animal experiments also confirmed the relationship between serum ACE activity and table salt in rats (Figure 19.3).

They reviewed the studied table salt synergism using plant fibers that can absorb either sodium or chlorine among table salt components to promote the excretion of sodium or chlorine in feces. When normal and hypertensive rats were raised for several weeks with high-salt feed

* *Renin:* A type of protease mainly secreted in the kidney of higher animals that is related with the rise in blood pressure. Abnormally high renin secretion leads to severe hypertension such as cardiovascular hypertension, malignant hypertension, and even hypertension due to renin-producing cytoma in rare cases.

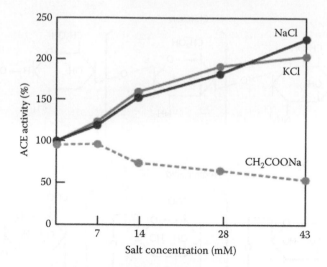

*Figure 19.2* ACE activation by sodium chloride.

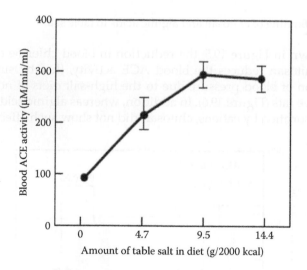

*Figure 19.3* Blood ACE activity and table salt intake.

containing 5% plant fibers (alginic acid, chitosan) in the structure shown in Figure 19.4, all experimental groups grew normally and chlorine excretion in feces increased in the chitosan administration group such that the blood chlorine concentration decreased.

Serum ACE activity when no salt was added was regarded to be 100.

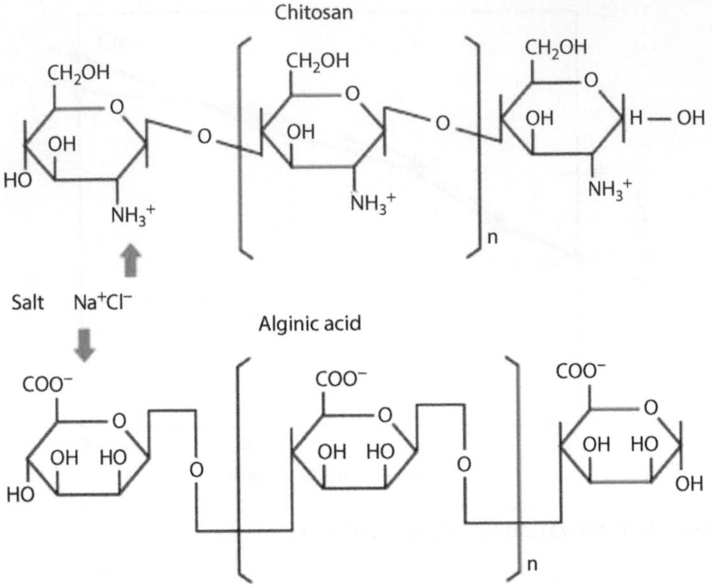

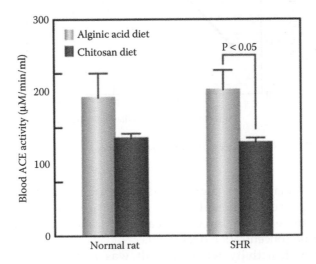

**Figure 19.4** Binding of chitosan and alginic acids to table salt.

As shown in Figure 19.5, the reduction in blood chlorine concentrations by chitosan reduces the blood ACE activity, thereby suppressing the elevation of blood pressure due to the high-salt diets of normal and hypertensive rats (Figure 19.6). In addition, whereas alginic acid inhibited mineral absorption by cations, chitosan did not show such effects.

**Figure 19.5** The effect of plant fibers on hypertension rats' ACE activity.

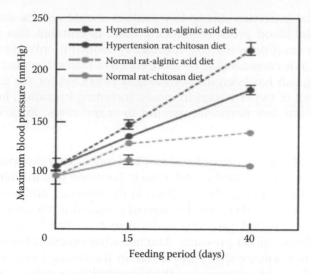

*Figure 19.6* Blood pressure-dropping effect of chitosan.

## 19.3 Clinical studies of the effects of chitosan on hypertension

When high-salt diets (table salt 13 g, 1,100 kcal/breakfast) were consumed by seven healthy males aged in the range between 20 and 55 years, elevation in the blood pressure appeared one hour later. However, when approximately 4 g of chitosan was orally administered simultaneously with high-salt diets for one week, the blood pressure elevation that occurred due to the high-salt diets disappeared, indicating that although the blood ACE elevated one hour after eating high-salt diets (because ACE was activated by chlorine), the elevation of ACE activity was inhibited by chitosan intake: in effect, the chitosan reduced the blood concentration of chlorine, thereby suppressing the elevation of blood pressure.

One interesting question to be explored is *what problems would occur if salt is unconditionally avoided for the reason that salt is not good for hypertension?*

In general, hypertension is a risk factor for stroke and, until now, it has been known that all hypertension-related diseases can be reduced by reducing the amount of salt in meals or sodium intake.

Recently, myocardial infarction was noted to occur at a high rate among male patients with hypertension who were being treated for such through low-sodium diets. Alderman et al. (1995) pointed out that low-sodium diets reduce the total blood volume, leading to an increase in blood viscosity, thereby reducing the blood volume in the coronary arteries. This consequently increased the risk of myocardial infarction. Although salt reduction is important in the treatment of hypertension, the complications of myocardial infarction due to low sodium should also be considered. Therefore, the blood pressure-reducing effect of chitosan that improves low sodium conditions thereby specifically reducing only chlorine that activates ACE is considered to be more effective than salt reduction.

Recently, salt has been unconditionally restricted for the prevention and treatment of hypertension in meals, including breakfast, lunch, and dinner, without any particular ground in many cases. Even when the same high-salt diet has been consumed, urine excretion of table salt differs with time. The amount of table salt excretion is larger after dinner compared with that following breakfast and lunch. This is opposite to the daily cycle rhythm of blood aldosterone (a hormone that inhibits sodium excretion in the kidney), which is high in the morning and low at night. Aldosterone, a mineral corticoid (a steroid involved in the metabolism of electrolytes and water), promotes sodium reabsorption in the kidney to indirectly elevate blood pressure. Another adrenocortical hormone, glucocorticoid (a hormone that plays a role in increasing blood sugar and relieving inflammation), increases the susceptibility of aldosterone. In the morning, when the blood concentrations (levels) of these two hormones rise, blood pressure is also prone to rise while performing activities, which is natural and necessary for the adaptation to living environments. If the rhythm of the hormones is normal, it is not necessary to restrict salt in all three meals per day but salt may be restricted in breakfast and lunch with high-blood aldosterone and may be relatively less restricted in dinner.

## 19.4   Obesity and hypertension

When humans become lean or weak, they tend to have low blood pressure. Similarly, the blood pressure in obese individuals increases in proportion to the degree of obesity. The causes of the rise in the blood pressure due to obesity include hyperinsulinism (a condition characterized by hypoglycemia due to excessive secretion of insulin from the pancreas) resulting from insulin resistance.

In obese people, the maximum blood pressure and serum insulin values have shown to have a clear correlation with each other.

When glucose tolerance tests (tests in which glucose is artificially loaded into the blood to analyze its utilization) are conducted in obese people with normal glucose tolerance (the glucose throughput of living bodies), the insulin secretion of those with hypertension increases more so than that of those with normal blood pressure. Therefore, those with obesity and hypertension can enhance blood pressure-reducing effects and improve insulin resistance through changes in diet and exercise.

In this respect, improving the hyperinsulinemia (the insulin resistance of obese people) is considered to be an effective method for the treatment of hypertension. Chlorine in table salt is involved in the foregoing

*Table 19.2* Insulin secretion and table salt components
of hypertension rats

|  | Blood insulin (μu/mL) |
| --- | --- |
| High sodium and chlorine diet | 88.6 ± 10.7 |
| High sodium diet(no chlorine) | 65.5 ± 7.29 |
| High chlorine diet(no sodium) | 80.9 ± 10.1 |

as a dietary factor that promotes insulin secretion. Kato et al. (2001) reported that blood chlorine concentrations and insulin secretion are correlated with each other (Table 19.2) such that chitosan can suppress not only insulin secretion but also the absorption of extra dietary fat by reducing the level of blood chlorine.

Table salt, which contains sodium and chlorine, is a trace nutrient that is involved in humoral regulation and the regulation of blood pressure. It also serves as a basic seasoning to improve taste. The chlorine in table salt activates the digestive enzymes that act on carbohydrates and proteins (amylase and pepsinogen), whereas sodium promotes the intestinal absorption of digestive products. Eventually, table salt plays particularly important roles in increasing appetite and in the digestion and absorption of food. However, if the dietary life of eating salty food is a habit, it may cause hypertension. Therefore, appropriate salt control is necessary for the maintenance of proper health and the prevention of diseases.

The role of involvement of table salt in blood pressure is still debatable. In particular, although scientific data demonstrating a direct association between chlorine and hypertension are rare, since sodium is consumed mostly in the form of sodium chloride, the epidemiological evidence for sodium intake in relation to hypertension is also considered in relation to chlorine intake and hypertension.

## 19.5 Development of antihypertensive materials from fish skin

To efficiently utilize fish skin, which is a fishery processing byproduct, we extracted collagen protein from Alaska pollack skin (which contains more than 80% collagen protein) and then decomposed the collagen protein using enzymes to synthesize low-molecular hydrolysates that can be absorbed into living bodies. The effects of the peptides isolated from these hydrolysates to inhibit ACE, which plays an important role in the regulation of the blood pressure, were measured. According to the results, the inhibitory concentration $(IC)_{50}$ value of the peptides (glycine-proline-leucine) isolated from the Alaska pollack skin degradation product was the lowest, indicating that the concentration that could inhibit ACE by 50%

**Table 19.3** The ACE inhibitory effects of the peptides isolated from fish protein hydrolysates

| Raw material | Peptide | $IC_{50}$(uM) |
|---|---|---|
| Alaska pollack skin collagen | Gly-Pro-Leu | 2.65 |
| Alaska pollack skin collagen | Gly-Pro-Met | 17.13 |
| Alaska pollack meat protein | Phe-Gly-Ala-Ser-Thr-Arg-Gly-Ala | 14.7 |
| Flatfish skin collagen | Met-lle-Phe-Pro-Gly-Ala-Gly-Gly-Pro-Glu-Leu | 10.75 |
| Flatfish meat protein | Arg-Pro-Asp-Phe-Asp-Leu-Glu-Pro-Pro-Try | 15.02 |

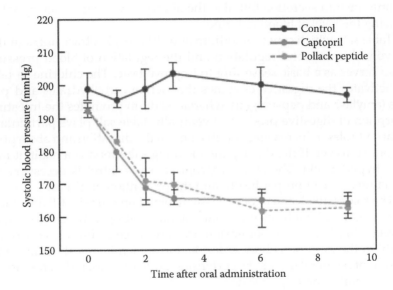

**Figure 19.7** Antihypertensive effect of Alaska pollack skin collagen hydrolysis peptide.

was 2.65 mm. This implies an efficient inhibitory effect of these peptides against ACE (Table 19.3).

Therefore, when the peptides (glycine-proline-leucine) were administered to the animal models of congenital hypertension and the antihypertensive effect was measured, the systolic blood pressure dropped by at least 30 mmHg in 2 h after administration. Moreover, blood pressure suppression effects similar to those of the commercially available antihypertensive captopril were demonstrated.

As such, fish skin, which is rarely utilized for other purposes than animal feed, can be developed into high-value-added products through simple processes (Figure 19.7).

# chapter twenty

# Fish oil is an adult disease preventive medicine

Dr. Crawford of the Institute of Brain Chemistry and Human Nutrition in the United Kingdom, once pointed out that the reason behind the high intelligence quotient of Japanese children is that they have been consuming food rich in fish from a young age (Crawford and Marsh, 2002). Therefore, in Japan, campaigns are conducted for the prevention of various diseases by the spread of fish meals under the catchphrase that if one eats fish, that they will become smarter.

With this in mind, *what in the fish is good for human bodies?* The nutrients indispensable for the proper growth of the human body should include proteins and various vitamins. However, fish has been found to be a very good source of food for health, particularly because of the presence of eicosapentaenoic acid (EPA) and docosahexaenoic acid (DHA), which constitute the main components of fish oil.

Studies on EPA date back to more than 30 years ago. In Japan, for the first time in the world, EPA from sardine oil purified up to 90% was put on the market as an obstructive arteriosclerosis therapeutic agent in 1990 because it was recognized to have platelet aggregation inhibitory effects. Currently, it has a market value exceeding $45.76 million, and is being evaluated as a drug with fewer side effects and can be easily utilized in clinical tests. In 1994, EPA was also recognized as having effects to reduce neutral fat and cholesterol. Additionally, it was approved for the indication of antihyperlipidemic agent by the Department of Health and Human Services of Japan. Therefore, it is expected to gain a further presence in the pharmaceutical market.

Although DHA is one of the major components of fish oil along with EPA, the research and development of DHA have been delayed because of the difficulty in the procurement of highly pure DHA for research purposes. However, as DHA is found in fish such as tuna and bonito, the necessary development has progressed rapidly in the last five years such that DHA was finally commercialized.

## 20.1   EPA production by marine microorganisms and genetic engineering

The discovery of microorganisms that produce EPA has led to its large-scale synthesis. Although EPA is the main component of fish oil, fish cannot synthesize EPA by themselves. EPA is contained in fish meat or fish oil because of the food chain, in which algae or plant planktons are the primary producers. Prior to 1986, the fact that microorganisms make EPA was hardly known.

In 1986, however, EPA-producing bacteria were successfully discovered from microorganisms that coexist in the intestines of external blue-colored fishes, such as horse mackerel, sardine, and mackerel, which contain large amounts of EPA in their oil. Although attempts were made to produce EPA as a medicinal formulation by mass-culturing of these bacteria, the production of EPA turned out to be disadvantageous as compared with of sardine oil in terms of production costs. Therefore, since EPA is produced by bacteria, genetic engineering methods that separate EPA to produce biosynthetic genes from the bacteria are currently being attempted for the mass production of EPA.

Genetic engineering involves manipulating these EPA-producing biosynthetic genes using organisms with no originality to produce EPA, such as seaweed or higher plants, for example. Although synthesis of EPA in large quantities at low costs in microorganisms suffers from limited productivity, if EPA can be produced by living organisms capable of producing large amounts of oils and fats, such as yeasts, mold, and algae, or from higher plants from which edible fats and oils can be collected, such as soybean and rapeseeds, new functional foods can be developed.

Although it is still a dream at this point, there are cases in which EPA biosynthetic genes have been isolated and utilized successfully to synthesize EPA in *Escherichia coli*, which is incapable of synthesizing EPA, by gene manipulation. In addition, there are cases in which EPA genes were introduced into blue-green algae to confer an EPA production capability. The time will come soon when vegetables, cereals, and fruits are manipulated genetically to synthesize EPA so that EPA that cannot be taken from other sources, such as fish and shellfish, can be easily taken.

The fatty acids of fish oils that have been known thus far are composed mostly of EPA. However, though the content of DHA is only a few percent in these fish, the composition of the fatty acids of tuna is completely opposite. Importantly, the orbital oil of tuna contains as much as 30% DHA (Table 20.1) and only contains 6% to 7% EPA.

Moreover, tuna heads are always disposed of as marine waste, and only an extremely small part is utilized as feed or fertilizer. The fatty oil is used as a boiler fuel in place of heavy oil. Therefore, the orbital oil of tuna and bonito may serve as potential raw materials for DHA. Since highly

*Table 20.1* DHA and EPA contents in marine fish orbital oils

| Marine fish (orbital oil) | DHA (%) | EPA (%) |
|---|---|---|
| Bigeye tuna | 30.6 | 7.8 |
| Bluefin tuna | 28.5 | 6.1 |
| Yellow tuna | 28.9 | 4.5 |
| Bonito | 42.5 | 9.5 |
| Spearfish | 28.4 | 3.9 |
| Swordfish | 9.6 | 3.4 |
| Yellowtail amberjack | 10.8 | 3.3 |
| Great amberjack | 20.5 | 6.5 |
| Horse mackerel | 15.3 | 15.3 |
| Sardine | 12.1 | 22.6 |
| Bullhead shark | 29.0 | 3.0 |
| Spotted dogfish | 12.5 | 13.4 |

pure DHA with a purity exceeding 99% used as a reagent is very expensive, amounting to approximately $70 for 100 mg, or $700 for 1 g, animal experiments and other research activities based on DHA could not be easily conducted. Therefore, DHA had to be extracted from orbital oil, and highly pure DHA could be obtained in large quantities at low prices by refining the DHA obtained from orbital oil, leading to rapid progress in the initiation of DHA studies.

In addition, this orbital oil can be sufficiently used as food because it is fresh and has no hygiene problem. Following the discovery of the fact that tuna orbital oil contains DHA at a high concentration, the development of food, especially dietary supplements, has been accelerated.

## 20.2 Pharmacological activity of DHA and switch to healthy food

DHA, an unsaturated fatty acid, is a food nutrient with diverse pharmacological actions, including the development of the nervous system, improvement of learning functions, improvement of retinal reflectance, anticancer activity, anti-allergic action, and lipid-lowering action. It can be considered an effective nutrient for the prevention of various adult diseases and a preventive medicinal functional health food with tertiary functions. In particular, DHA is fundamentally different from EPA in that it can pass the blood-brain barrier.*

---

* *Blood-brain barrier:* The functional barrier that exists between blood circulation and the brain and that is specific for the passage of substances.

DHA is involved in nerve and memory/learning functions, which cannot be expected from EPA. Currently, a considerable action mechanism of DHA has been revealed, and clinical trials of DHA in humans have proven that its use leads to an improvement of senile dementia. Similar to other important pharmacological actions, an improvement of atopic dermatitis has also been demonstrated, and the revelation of diverse effects, such as the prevention of occurrence and metastasis of cancers, reduction of blood cholesterol, and suppression of a rise in blood pressure, has also occurred.

In addition, the development of healthy foods supplemented with DHA-containing fats and oils has rapidly progressed recently. The market of such healthy foods has grown into a large revenue exceeding ¥50 billion in Japan. The market is expected to be expanded further with the advancement of various technologies, such as those involving antioxidative activity, stability, pulverization, and emulsification of DHA.

The production of tuna in South Korea is 221,000 tons per year. Out of this total production, 51,000 tons are used as raw materials for canning, which accounts for approximately 81% of the entire canned food production; 63,000 tons constitutes fish and shellfish. Since several thousand tons of the heads, intestines, and bones are discarded when tuna is processed every year, we hope to utilize these waste products and convert them into functional materials that can prevent adult diseases.

## 20.3   Senile dementia-improving effect

Dementia, which we commonly call senility, etymologically means being out of one's mind, or characterized by a frantic state of mind. Although it has been regarded to be a natural physiological phenomenon that occurs due to aging, it is clearly a nervous system disease that presents due to the development of degenerative lesions in the brain. Dementia, a clinical syndrome, which commonly occurs in elderly people aged 65 years or more, causes encumbrances in work-life, social activities, and interpersonal relationships with disabilities in mental functions, such as memory, judgment, and the ability to think. It may result due to damage to the brain by external injuries, cerebrovascular disorders, or various metabolic disorders even before the age of 65 years. Former president of the United States, Ronald Reagan, did not even know that he was the president due to having Alzheimer's disease, the most common form of dementia. It surprised people worldwide and resulted in family feuds. Dementia is also emerging as a serious social problem in South Korea.

However, it has been found that the administration of DHA, an unsaturated fatty acid, present in large amounts in fish, relieves senile dementia. The fact that DHA administration improves brain functions has been demonstrated long ago in experiments using animals and, recently, it has been reported to procure excellent results in improving human brain function.

For instance, Japanese media reported that in Japan, a clinical trial on the effects of DHA on brain function improvement was conducted on 13 patients with dementia and five patients with Alzheimer's disease in the hospital who were aged between 57 and 94 years. Upon oral administration of 10 to 20 DHA capsules (70 mg per capsule) every day for six months, 10 out of 13 cerebrovascular dementia patients reported a stronger will to live with fewer delusions. The five patients with Alzheimer's disease had a slightly improved will to live, with an improvement to some extent in interpersonal relations and in the maintenance of composure.

The results of indirect tests of intellectual functions indicated that patients not administered with DHA had brain functions that declined slowly, while those administered with DHA demonstrated effects that improved their calculation ability and judgment in six months. In addition, there was no side effects except for stomachache, which occurred in patients due to an excessive intake of fats.

The related research team claims that after its entry into the brains of patients with dementia, which occurs because of the dead nerve cells in the brain, DHA activates the living nerve cells, thereby making them functionally active. Therefore, DHA can be regarded to be effective for the improvement and prevention of dementia, although it cannot be considered as a fundamental remedy for dementia. The increase in senile dementia in Japan is related with the noted change in dietary life from a diet centered on fish (protein-rich diet) to one centered on meat (fat-rich diet). Dementia-related symptoms seem to have increased in South Korea, too, where the consumption of meat-centered diets have witnessed a recent surge.

In addition to dementia-improving effects, some clinical results demonstrated an improvement rate of 50% in pediatric patients with atopic dermatitis with the use of DHA. Many other clinical trials are in progress. Hereafter, the usefulness and effectiveness of DHA are expected to be proved through more reliable study results.

## chapter twenty-one

# Development of an ointment from sea cucumber extract for treatment of athlete's foot

## 21.1  Identity of molds

Molds and humans have deep connections with each other dating back to the old days. For instance, wine, soybean paste, and soy sauce are made by molds through fermentation. Some of the components made by molds have been recently developed into numerous antibiotics such as penicillin that now greatly help human beings to treat various diseases in real life or otherwise. On the other hand, mold is also considered a *villain* that damages food, clothes, and shoes, thereby causing harm to humans. Molds growing inside nuclear reactors, which are completely filled with radioactive substances, also become a cause of the trouble. Above all, diseases caused by the propagation of molds inside the human body are directly harmful to human health. Harmful molds that cause diseases are very tenacious, such as the ones that remain attached to food or clothes and hardly get detached. The absence of drugs that are effective on such disease-causing molds necessitates many efforts for treatment.

Recently, more and more species of molds are becoming tolerant to drugs such as antibiotics and adrenocortical hormones, which are used to strongly suppress bacterial infections, thereby making the treatment of mold diseases more difficult. The above-mentioned phenomenon, called *superinfection,* even leads to cases in which species of molds such as *Aspergillus* and *Mucor* that are normally not harmful to the human body and used for preparing rice, cakes, and bread, break inside the human lungs and other internal organs, resulting in death. In addition, ringworm and athlete's foot are among other well-known mold diseases that invade the skin. The cases of infection caused by the fungus *Candida albicans*, which is similar to yeast and which invades the fingers of housewives who carry out household tasks such as cooking or washing, have also been increasing in number. The picture of a sea cucumber is shown in Figure 21.1.

---

* *Superinfection*: Infection of cells or entities, which are already infected with a species of pathogen again by homologous or heterologous pathogens.

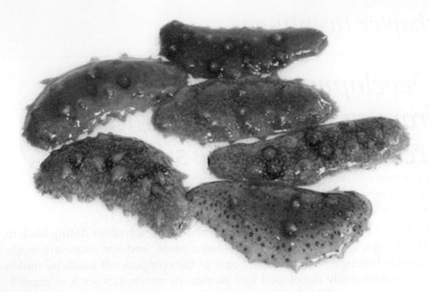

*Figure 21.1* A picture of a sea cucumber.

The various conditions that are necessary for microorganisms, including molds, bacteria, and viruses, to invade the human body and cause diseases are called *infection factors*. The above-mentioned conditions can be of two types: conditions of the invading germs and socio-environmental conditions. Diseases do not develop even after the invasion of germs into the human body unless the above-mentioned conditions are met to some extent.

Germs can be classified into pathogens and nonpathogens. Pathogens are highly toxic and always prompt certain symptoms while invading the human body to cause diseases. The pathogenic species of molds that cause infection in animals are, in general, highly toxic, and they tend to be fatal to the human body. A typical skin disease caused by molds in humans is athlete's foot. Mold infections are closely related with social and environmental conditions, and such relationships can be evidenced by the fact that athlete's foot is more common in civilized countries and in cities than in farming areas. In fact, 30% to 90% of urban populations suffer from athlete's foot disease.

For instance, molds can easily proliferate in white-collar workers who commute on the subway trains that carry passengers in the morning and evening, because white-collar workers wear a tie and a shirt even in the summer and always wear shoes in their offices. Furthermore, although safety shoes should be mandatorily worn in factories for preventing dangers, such shoes are not breathable at all and can be said to be *extremely hazardous* with regard to the onset of athlete's foot. In addition, a hot and humid environment cannot be avoided inside steel mills and coal mines. In fact, individuals who work in such places are said to be more highly prone to having athlete's foot than those who work elsewhere. Workplaces and also homes have been recently equipped with room heating facilities so that people can stay protected from the cold in winter. Therefore, even in midwinter, cases of athlete's foot increasingly appear in the same way as they do in midsummer.

In general, athlete's foot and climate are closely related to each other. The number of athlete's foot patients increases when the temperature exceeds 15°C and humidity exceeds 70% but decreases when either of these two conditions are absent. Therefore, athlete's foot disease will not occur unless both the conditions of high temperature and high humidity are satisfied. However, athlete's foot is bound to torment human beings further as the earth's temperature is expected to increase continuously due to the phenomenon of El Niño.

Athlete's foot refers to a disease that appears on the skin, nails, and hair when dermatophytes, a type of mold, become parasitic on the stratum corneum of the skin. In fact, athlete's foot can occur anywhere on the skin and can be classified according to their site of occurrence into head athlete's foot, body athlete's foot, dhobi itch (groin), beard athlete's foot, facial athlete's foot, hand athlete's foot, and foot athlete's foot, respectively. Among them, foot athlete's foot, which is the most common and accounts for approximately 40% of all cases of athlete's foot, is further classified into interdigital types in which the interdigital regions fester, cornification types in which subjective symptoms are hardly shown, and vesicular types in which many small blisters appear on the sole and sides of the foot, thereby making the affected regions quite itchy. In many cases, different types of athlete's foot occur in combination with each other. Foot athlete's foot gets transmitted as the fungi (molds) present in the keratin separated from patients infect others in crowded places such as bathhouses, swimming pools, Korean dry sauna baths, and so on, through fine wounds on the feet. Feet can easily get infected because they sweat a lot, become sweaty when well-ventilated shoes are not worn, and often have damage to the skin caused by mechanical stimulation due to walking.

Nail athlete's foot accounts for 50% of all nail diseases and its prevalence increases with age as normal immune functions decline. On the other hand, the prevalence of diabetes and peripheral vascular disease increases with age. Nails in the toes are between four and 10 times more frequently infected than nails in the fingers. Although 90% of nail athlete's foot cases are caused by dermatophytes, about one-third of cases of nail athlete's foot occurring on the fingernails are caused by a yeast fungus named *Candida*. In most cases, toenail athlete's foot occurs when foot athlete's foot is neglected so that dermatophytes are able to spread to the toenails. On the other hand, fingernail athlete's foot occurs in some cases, when toenail athlete's foot is very severe that dermatophytes spread to fingernails. Fingernail athlete's foot is also caused by *Candida*, mainly in people who work with water.

Nail athlete's foot is not only ugly but also a source of secondary infection because this disease infects other body parts of the patient and other individuals. The affected nails gradually bend and thicken so that they cannot be easily cut, grow into the flesh, and cause inconvenience during walking. Furthermore, pain can occur, inflammation can be induced in the soft tissues, or the self-esteem of the patient may be lowered, thereby causing encumbrances to social life. Athlete's foot, which occurs in areas other than the feet, is characterized by erythematous lesions accompanied by circular or semicircular dead skin cells with clear boundaries that spread efferently. Papules (small rashes appearing on the skin), small blisters, and pustules are also found to occur at the boundaries. Keratinization and hyperpigmentation occur as lesions as the boundaries gradually become larger and the lesions at the center are cured. Dhobi itch, which commonly occurs in adult males, is aggravated in the summer and, in many cases, only demonstrates pigmented spots in the winter. Head athlete's foot was common between the 1950s and 1970s but is now a rare disease, mainly occurring in school-age children. After invading the stratum corneum of the scalp, the fungi (molds) propagate themselves downward along hair follicles, leading to hair loss or breakage and causing very severe inflammation. A substance contained in sea cucumbers has been recently found to kill dermatophytes and is being utilized as a remedy for athlete's foot in Japan.

## 21.2   Components of athlete's foot ointment in sea cucumbers

Sea cucumbers were originally called *sea ginseng* and are literally used in medicine like ginseng has been widely used for cooking and as a tonic food. In addition to being a food rich in proteins, calcium, phosphorus, and iron, sea cucumbers stimulate appetite, assist metabolism, and are effective for preventing obesity because they are low in calories. Dried sea cucumbers that are consumed in the summer are better in taste and nutrition than raw sea cucumbers (also called *winter solstice sea cucumbers*) that are consumed in the winter. The iodine concentration increases when sea cucumbers are dried and consumption of such dried sea cucumbers can strengthen the heart. Dried sea cucumbers can be eaten either by boiling them so that they can be easily digested or after immersing them in water. Furthermore, the consumption of dried sea cucumbers after soaking in them water and with the addition of vinegar are effective for treating hypertension.

Sea cucumbers can prevent aging of the skin and blood vessels, including arteriosclerosis. Moreover, they are effective against cancer and gastric ulcer because they have a component called chondroitin sulfuric acid. Sea cucumbers can prevent/treat anemia and can also smooth liver movements because they not only have components such as calcium and tannin but also contain large amounts of taurine, which is a component of bile.

Although the beginning of using sea cucumbers as a food is unclear, a story about sea cucumbers in early Japanese records from the eighth century indicates that sea cucumbers closely coexisted with the people of Japan since prehistoric times. The lower bills, on which the words *dried sea cucumber* were written on the wooden tablets discovered in the Heijojyo ruins, indicated that dried sea cucumbers were sent to the Yamato Court as a specialty of the province.

Sea cucumbers appeared in ancient literature as *sea rats* or *sea ginseng*. Among the contents pertaining to the medicinal uses of sea cucumbers, particularly in relation with athlete's foot, the *Compendium of Materia Medica* has a record that suggests that if a dried powder made of sea cucumbers is applied on to the surfaces of purulent wounds, that the wounds will be cleaned such that they could be cured. In addition, the *Compendium of Foods* has a record, indicating that *ringworm of the scalp* can be cured by attaching sea cucumber slices cut much like thick paper (made by cutting live sea cucumbers after removing their internal organs) by opening them to the affected areas on the scalp. The above-mentioned records suggest that sea cucumbers not only have a factor that promotes the regeneration of tissues but also contain components in their bodies that are effective against athlete's foot.

Studies have been conducted for determining the effectiveness of sea cucumber extract against athlete's foot considering the verbal records, which indicated that upon boiling, sea cucumber extract is effective against athlete's foot, and also with respect to the stories of experiences in treating athlete's foot using sea cucumbers and treatment progression. As a result, a substance called holotoxin that can kill molds was identified in sea cucumbers. Holotoxin, a saponin glycoside, is a complex consisting of three components: holotoxin A, holotoxin B, and holotoxin C. In addition, the tertiary structure of the sugar chain part has been known to play an important role in the expression of anti-mold activities of holotoxins. The results of clinical tests conducted by the Holosri Co. in Japan, using the tertiary structure of the sugar chain part, showed that 86.3% of sea cucumber samples were effective with 29.5% of samples remarkably effective, 49.6% of samples effective, and 7.2% of samples slightly effective, thereby indicating that only 13.7% of samples were ineffective.

The high rates of effectiveness of sea cucumber extract were also recognized by diseases as the ratios of cases, where 83.8% of *slightly effective* or *more effective* sea cucumber samples were for athlete's foot, 91.3% of samples were for dhobi itch, 75.0% of samples were for cutaneous candidiasis, 100.0% of samples were for interdigital blastomycotic caused by *Candida*, 100.0% of samples were for tinea versicolor, and 100.0% of samples were for white comb.

Altogether, nine side effects were recognized that included stimulation, blush, dermatitis, pain, boil, and itch, with an expression rate of 9.5%. According to some studies, synthetic holotoxins could be used as drugs with less stimulation and side effects. In addition, holotoxins showed sufficient treatment effects, despite their concentrations being much lower in comparison with the remedial agents used against general athlete's foot. Furthermore, *Trichophyton* did not acquire drug resistance, considering that treatment effects did not decline even when holotoxins were used for longer periods of time. Thus, even when applied externally, holotoxins are known to effectively treat fingernail athlete's foot.

Although the specificity of holotoxins cannot be attributed to the specificity of the chemical structure of saponin as such, holotoxins are complexly related not only to the physiology of *Trichophyton* but also to the physiology of the human body. Hence, it may be concluded that the discovery of the relationship between sea cucumbers and athlete's foot by our ancestors through experience is simply marvelous.

# chapter twenty-two

# Anti-aging effects of fish with high nucleic acid content such as sardine

## 22.1  Process of generation of the human body

As we grow older, the skin becomes dry and dull; wrinkles on the skin increase; the skin color becomes darker; the elasticity of the face disappears; and the skin of the eyelids, the cheek, and the chin begin to sag and loosen. Additionally, the hair becomes thin, the forehead becomes wrinkled, the hair on the forehead is lost, and gray hair begins to appear gradually. The phenomenon of aging that takes place in the human body begins to be realized when these phenomena occur in the body, regardless of our like or dislike. However, the reasons behind the occurrence of such a phenomenon should be known. The human body consists of 60 trillion cells. The entire human skin, muscles, heart, brain, eyes, hair, fingernails, and toenails are aggregates of cells. The different kinds of cells that make up the human body, such as the soft cells of the skin and the hard cells of the fingernails and toenails, respectively are similar in that they are all cells.

The human body undergoes aging due to the concomitant aging of the cells. So, *why do cells undergo aging?* The process through which the human body is generated must be briefly examined before understanding the concept of aging. The human body is generated from a fertilized egg cell or a zygote in which the sperm and the egg have been united into a single cell. When seen biologically, the growth of the human body is said to end in 20 years. However, a phenomenal vitality is shown by the single fertilized egg cell that divides itself to form 60 trillion cells in 20 years.

Deoxyribonucleic acid (DNA) governs cell division as such, creating the cells and proteins that are necessary for the human body to exist. Thus, nucleic acid controls the human body from the time of birth until the time of death. The total length of 1,000 cells arranged in a row will not even be 1 cm, since a typical cell is a small ball of approximately 10 µm in diameter, with a nucleus at the center that measures approximately one-quarter of the cell. The centrally located nucleus contains the nucleic acid called DNA—arguably the most important substance present in all cells across 1.35 million species of living organisms on Earth, including humans, cattle, rats, fish, insects, and microorganisms. As people grow older, something goes wrong in their heart, liver, bronchi of the lungs, and blood pressure such that they become more susceptible to contracting diseases. The above-mentioned association between the phenomenon of aging and the presence of DNA within the nuclei of cells can be easily seen if the two roles that are played by DNA are understood. The first role of DNA is to produce the same DNA molecule through the process of DNA replication that occurs inside the nucleus prior to cell division. The new daughter nucleus, formed by the division of the old nucleus, creates new cells as determined by the DNA transmitted into it. During the process of the generation of new living organisms, cells continuously divide and give rise to the new body in a process in which old cells are replaced by new cells. Usually, DNA replicates itself accurately. However, *what would happen if this DNA replication fails even a slight amount?*

DNA has a hand in everything related with cell structure and function. If a cell containing deformed DNA is a reproductive cell (a sperm or an ovum), then the offspring may be born as a congenitally deformed child. However, if the deformed DNA is not present in a reproductive cell but is present in a skin or a liver cell, then the new skin or liver cells produced by the incomplete DNA command will also be incomplete. Sometimes, this incompleteness appears in apparent forms such as cancer cells, but is seen more frequently in vague forms such as hypofunction, aging of the skin or hair, or damage to the liver and the heart.

The second role of DNA is the production of proteins. All parts of the human body, including the heart, the blood, and the skin, are mainly composed of proteins. The synthesis of these proteins is solely assigned to DNA, which, by combining amino acids (components of proteins) and with the help of ribonucleic acid (RNA), make proteins. Amino acid sequences of the newly synthesized proteins follow the instructions of genetic information already contained in the DNA molecule.

## 22.2   Causes of aging

Complete proteins cannot be synthesized if DNA fails, no matter how slight the failure is. As a result, such incompletely synthesized proteins become components of the human body in their incomplete states. In addition, the loss or decline of DNA function slows down the rate of protein synthesis, leading to the degeneration and loss of cells of the skin, hair, and internal organs, which cannot be easily recovered. Therefore, the phenomena of aging and chronic adult diseases occur in humans, as mentioned earlier. Among the diverse causes leading to the decline of DNA function, DNA damage is brought about by external factors such as viruses, X-rays, cosmic rays, and, in some cases, poisons. However, instead of such special cases, general damage to the DNA that can be experienced by anybody will be addressed here.

In considering the mechanism of damage to DNA, it should be asked, *why is the skin of youths healthy and beautifully shining and their hair glossy and attractive?* The rate of cell division is high in young people and proteins are continuously synthesized during the growth period of humans (until up to 20 years after birth), in line with cell division, because the two types of nucleic acids, DNA and RNA, are abundant and act vigorously. More importantly, these lively, youthful, healthy nucleic acids seldom fail to synthesize new cells or proteins. In fact, the human body can continue to live without undergoing any damage if the functions of these nucleic acids do not decline. However, humans are destined to grow older year by year and finally die.

With this in mind, *when do the lively nucleic acids lose their functions?* Nucleic acids are synthesized in the body, using proteins and carbohydrates. Certainly, nucleic acids can be synthesized to the extent that they are more than sufficient for use during the growth period of humans until the age of 20 years. However, the ability of the human body to synthesize nucleic acids declines extremely after the growth period ends. Cell division or protein production can hardly be accomplished with only the nucleic acids that are synthesized in the body. The newly synthesized DNA becomes incomplete if the amounts of nucleotides are absolutely insufficient and, as a result, poor quality cells are gradually made.

Wounds obtained during a young age are easily healed and, in many cases, completely disappear unless they are large or deep. Generally, young people are cured of physical injuries quickly, even when they suffer a fracture. However, wounds or fractures do not mend as quickly as people grow older, and traces of their wounds often remain in later years because the body declines with age. Consequently, the quality of nucleic acids also decreases and damaged or wounded cells in the body are no longer regenerated.

Conversely, it can be said that most wounds occur in the body after the age of 20 years because the ability of nucleic acids declines and, as a result, normal and healthy cells or appropriate amounts of proteins are not synthesized. Although the phenomenon of aging and most cases of chronic diseases cannot be explained solely by the decline in the ability of nucleic acids, the declining ability of nucleic acids is undoubtedly related to the phenomenon of aging.

## 22.3    Prevention of aging

The mechanism of aging has been gradually revealed and methods of prevention of aging have been published, despite the fact that aging over time cannot be avoided.

Nucleic acids are always present inside the cells of all living organisms and are supplied by food. Therefore, if humans always have fresh nucleic acids, similar to those present before the age of 20 years, then the human body should have no reason to decline. Thus, it could be worth considering, *what in the world might be good to take nucleic acids from?* However, nutritionists believe that humans are not required to take nucleic acids actively from the outside because sufficient amounts of nucleic acids are synthesized within the human body. Food items that contain huge amounts of nucleic acids are excluded probably for the reason that the components of nucleic acids, adenine, and guanine will increase the concentration of uric acid in the body, thereby causing gout and kidney stones. However, the normal functions of healthy, active cells prevent aging and bring about youthfulness. Therefore, nucleic acids are not nutrients that need to be ingested but rather are nutrients that must be actively ingested.

Nucleic acids are present inside the cells of all living organisms. The actual length of a DNA molecule inside a human cell is 174 cm, and the length of DNA molecules is different among different species of living organisms. For instance, the length of a DNA molecule is 77.5 cm in chicken, 198 cm in cows, and 1,683 cm in onions, respectively. In other words, the content of nucleic acids in a cell has already been determined based on the species of living organism. It should be noted here that foods with low nucleic acid content are eggs and milk, in which the nucleic acid content is close to nil. However, the nucleic acid content is never low in chickens and cows. An egg is a huge cell that contains nucleic acids corresponding to just a single cell. Milk does not contain any nucleic acids because milk is not a cell but a secretion, and nucleic acids are only present in cells. Foods with high nucleic acid content should be eaten for effective intake of nucleic acids. Eating foods with low nucleic acid content is not at all beneficial, no matter how many cells are taken in, because it may lead to excess calorie intake.

A special measuring instrument is not needed to test the fitness of aged people in comparison to those in their 20s because this can be checked simply by them going upstairs in a building, stepping on one of every two stairs. Old people typically still feel young if they are able to go up the stairs by approximately two floors without loss of breath. On the other hand, loss of breath and difficulty in body movements indicate a clear decline in pulmonary function. Breathing becomes difficult as pulmonary function declines with age. As a result, people feel uncomfortable and the phenomenon of oxygen deficiency occurs in each and every cell of the body as people grow older. Since cells require oxygen during energy generation, energy will naturally decrease if oxygen is not sufficiently supplied, leading to the vicious cycle of accelerated aging.

However, the intake of nucleic acids enables the cells in the body to carry out and maintain sufficient activities with less oxygen requirement.

In other words, nucleic acid therapy does not directly restore breathing function in humans but helps to utilize inhaled oxygen more effectively. The above-mentioned fact was also proved through experiments in rats, when a group of seven rats was raised on a nucleic acid-rich diet and another group of seven rats was raised on a normal diet. The animals were kept in glass bottles (one rat in each bottle), followed by sealing the bottles and recording the lengths of time of survival of the rats. Consequently, the rats belonging to the nucleic acid-rich diet intake group lived 48% longer and moved more actively than the rats belonging to the other group. Although there was one rat in the nucleic acid-rich diet intake group that did not move actively like the other rats, it lived twice as long as the rats that were not raised on a nucleic acid-rich diet.

As shown in Table 22.1, the nucleic acid content is high in fish. Nucleic acids contained in fish do not play the role of nucleic acids in the human body once they have been taken in, but are decomposed to become components during the synthesis of nucleic acids in humans. Similarly, proteins taken in by humans are decomposed into amino acids, which are absorbed and used as raw materials for protein synthesis in the human body.

*Table 22.1* Nucleic acid contents of foods

| Name of food | Content (mg/100 g) |
| --- | --- |
| Sardine (canned) | 590 |
| Chicken liver | 402[a] |
| Sardine (fish) | 343 |
| Anchovy | 341 |
| Salmon | 289 |
| Bovine liver | 268[a] |
| Hog liver | 259[a] |
| Oyster (canned) | 239[a] |
| Mackerel (fish) | 203 |
| Pea | 173 |
| Squid | 100[a] |
| Calf's liver | 88[a] |
| Hard clams | 85[a] |
| Flatfish | 82 |
| Bovine brain | 61[a] |

[a]  Nucleic acid content per 100 g of food (unit: mg) and Foods with high cholesterol values but that are rich in important nutrients.

## 22.4  *Effect of nucleic acids on the treatment of arthritis*

Benjamin Planck, MD, a prominent physician in the United States, reported that the administration of nucleic acids extracted from sardines in arthritis patients fundamentally cured arthritis because its recurrence was prevented. A sardine weighing 112 g contains at least 0.6 g of nucleic acids. In addition, sardine is rich in various vitamins that help nucleic acids carry out their activities. Sardine also contains minerals such as vanadium that lowers blood cholesterol values but can never be obtained from animal sources.

People living near the seashores of countries such as South Korea and Japan lead a long life, probably because they eat a lot of fish and sea algae. Eating plenty of fish such as sardines, anchovies, mackerels, and so on, and sea algae, may be a key to preventing aging and increasing longevity. People will be able to live longer if they live with proper exercise and positive ways of thinking.

# chapter twenty-three

# *Abundance of taurine in shellfishes*

## 23.1   *Efficacy of taurine*

Hippocrates, who is known as the father of medicine, in 400 BC mentioned that diseases could be healed by food and that the selection of appropriate foods would lead to the way to health. As the roles of these nutrients in the body are diverse and organically related with each other, if even only one nutrient is in excess or is deficient, then the nutritional balance will be hampered, causing damage to health. Therefore, if the knowledge of proper food and nutrition is actively reflected on the daily diet, many people can prevent foodborne diseases and maintain health. Therefore, South Korea and other countries in the world are aiming to identify physiological functional components that have not yet been revealed among the components present in foods.

Among them, taurine, present abundantly specifically in fish and shellfish among all marine products, has attracted global attention, owing to its physiological activity revealed recently. Taurine became known after its isolation from ox bile in 1827 by Tiedemann and Gmelin. Taurine is a type of amino acid that is present in large quantities in octopus, squid, shrimp, and shellfishes. The amounts of taurine in 100 g of the edible portion are 1,670.0 mg in octopus, 2,449.6 mg in Chinese mitten crab, 341.6 mg in squid, 630 mg in worm shell, 1,660 mg in cockle, 400 mg in sea cucumber, 1,080 mg in hard clam, and 1,080 mg in an oyster, respectively.

Taurine is also produced in an extremely small quantity in the human body. Therefore, taurine is probably an essential amino acid for children and the elderly. Originally, taurine (β-aminoethane sulfonate) is an amino acid derivative with a molecular weight of 125.14 Da, in which the carboxyl group (−COOH) in the amino acid structure is substituted by a sulfonyl group (−SO$_3$H). Although usually amino acids refer to amino carboxylic acids, because the metabolism of amino sulfonic acids in the human body is similar to that of amino carboxylic acids, taurine has been also called an amino acid. Taurine is a colorless, columnar crystalline compound with a melting point of 240°C ± 0.5°C. It is neutral in aqueous solutions because it is present as a salt (⁺H$_3$N-CH$_2$CH$_2$-SO$_3$⁻), is water-soluble, and is hardly soluble in ethanol and ether.

Although taurine was discovered more than 170 years ago, its physiological actions known were osmoregulation in marine animals, energy for muscle contraction in annelids, and bile acid generation in higher animals. However, since the mid-1980s, studies have reported that taurine is effective in adult diseases such as arteriosclerosis, hypertension, stroke, and heart failure; therefore, it can be said that the importance of taurine has been rediscovered, as the effects observed on such adult diseases can be found to stem from the peculiar physiological actions of taurine.

The representative physiological actions of taurine include bile acid production, cholesterol regulation, cell membrane ion transport regulation, antioxidation, and neurotransmission. Taurine, which is abundantly present in the colostrum of animals, is contained in almost all tissues in mammals. It is present at high concentrations in tissues of vital organs rather than in body fluids, particularly in the heart, skeletal muscles, brain, and genitals. In general, cats are animals that cannot biosynthesize taurine. In a cat raised on feed without taurine, the retina will degenerate soon and the cat will become completely blind in several weeks. Therefore, cats deprived of taurine prey on mice to supplement insufficient levels of taurine. These facts indicate the important roles of taurine in living beings for maintaining physiological functions.

Taurine is always maintained at a constant concentration in a healthy body, but its dynamic state in the body changes when the body is stimulated or disturbed. Under conditions of stress, infection by bacteria, surgery, injury, exposure to radiation, or excessive alcohol consumption, the amount of taurine excreted in the urine increases drastically, up to two to four times that excreted at normal conditions. Eventually, the amount of taurine in the body is reduced and the physiological balance controlled by taurine is hampered, leading to various diseases. In such situations, the amount of taurine to be supplemented externally to recover the physiological balance is approximately 200 to 1,000 mg, and if an individual suffers from a disease, at least 1,000 mg per day of taurine will be necessary, depending on the disease present. Therefore, frequently consuming fish and shellfish with high taurine contents will help to overcome stimulation from disturbance due to external factors or to prevent and treat adult diseases due to aging.

## 23.2    Cardioprotective action

In cardiac cells, taurine exists at a high concentration, and the content of taurine is the second highest among amino acids. If calcium ions that determine myocardial contractility are insufficient, the contraction of the heart will occur insufficiently. This will lead to conditions similar to congestive heart failure,* in which blood remains in the heart, and if calcium ions are in excess, the heart will contract excessively, causing damage to myocardial cells. Taurine plays the role of a regulator that regulates the calcium ion concentration in the heart. When calcium ions are at the normal physiological concentration, taurine has no effect on heart contraction. However, when the calcium ion concentration is below the normal concentration, taurine reduces myocardial contractility to control the contraction of the heart. Taurine has been reported as a cardiotonic drug.[†] The Italian National Formulary (Anno) contains taurine 500 mg capsules as a drug effective for angina, myocardial infarction, and chronic coronary heart diseases; these capsules are commercially available in Italy.

## 23.3    Effects on hypertension

Taurine lowered the blood pressure in white rats in which hypertension occurred naturally, but did not lower the blood pressure in normal white rats. This effect also appears in essential hypertension patients. The activity of cysteine dioxygenase declined and the taurine concentration reduced in the brains of white rats in which hypertension occurred naturally. In addition, taurine improves lipid or cholesterol metabolism and is effective for preventing arteriosclerosis or thrombosis.

## 23.4    Bile acid detoxification effect

Of the bile acids biosynthesized from cholesterol in the liver, lithocholic acid, among primary bile acids such as cholic acid and deoxycholic acid, forms polymers with glycine or taurine before being secreted as bile. Glycine or taurine forms a polymer with bile acid to accelerate fat absorption in the intestine. However, a more important reason is to detoxify bile acids. Taurine polymers are studied as a bile acid antidote because they have been found to be higher in quantity and lower in toxicity.

## 23.5    Removal of toxic substances in cells

Taurine is present at very high concentrations in cells or tissues where oxides can be easily generated, such as in the retina and neutrophils. In the retina, various types of oxides can be easily generated by the

---

* *Congestive heart failure*: A disease characterized by the decline of heart functions leading to difficulty in breathing, edema, and an abnormal accumulation of salt and water.
† *Cardiotonic drug*: A drug used in the treatment of heart failure, a condition in which the heart is unable to supply enough blood for organ tissues in the body.

actions of light and enzymes and, in neutrophils, oxides are generated by enzymes during phagocytosis. Living beings require low molecular scavengers, and taurine successfully plays the role of a scavenger.

Oxygen and nitrogen oxides, which are pollutants, cause many health problems by prompting damage to the lungs. Lung damage can be prevented by taurine administration. This preventive effect of taurine was confirmed in animal experiments in which animals were treated with ozone, which is an oxygen oxide. The preventive effect appears to happen because taurine removes free radicals, which are oxidants before they react with cell membranes.

## 23.6   Defense against lung damage by pollution

Modern people are at a higher risk than their ancestors of being exposed to a severely contaminated atmosphere, which can damage their lungs following subjection to oxidizing pollutants. Ozone and nitrite gases are representative pollutants and strong oxidants and, in particular, ozone is a major component of smog. Both destroy the epidermal cells of the airway and lungs and the endothelial cells of capillary vessels in tissues when inhaled into the human body through the airway, resulting in bronchial edema and hypertrophy. In such events, immunocytes (macrophages and polymorphonuclear neutrophils) in the surroundings gather and activate to defend the cells. The activated immunocytes secrete inflammation mediators and harmful oxygen species with tremendous destructive power. The harmful oxygen species destroy the cells more severely, leading to the amplification of the inflammatory responses of the bronchi and lungs.

Schuller-Levis et al. (1994) showed that taurine effectively protects against lung damage caused by pollutants such as ozone. To investigate whether taurine has protective effects, the authors confined rats administered with taurine and rats not administered with taurine in enclosed spaces, made them inhale ozone, extracted their lungs, and examined the lung tissues. Damage to the lungs was remarkably less in the rats administered with taurine than in the rats not administered with taurine. Although harmful oxygen species are unceasingly generated at normal conditions because of metabolic processes, the species are quickly removed normally as enzymes and physiological substances that clear them away are present in the body. However, when the amount of oxides inhaled from outside is large, the lung tissues will be destroyed if the treatment capacity of the tissues is exceeded. Taurine has been shown to change into taurine chloride in the lungs and inhibit the generation of harmful oxygen species.

In experiments conducted using human lung epidermal cells, Cantin clearly demonstrated that taurine protects the lungs from the toxicity of harmful oxygen species. He measured the amount of taurine required to remove harmful oxygen species from human lung epidermal cells. Based on the results, he found that when the amount of harmful oxygen species in cells increased because of the inhalation of pollutants, more taurine would be required than that required under normal conditions, and that toxicity would be exacerbated when the amount of taurine was insufficient.

Melanie et al. (1990) reported identical results in experiments conducted using the lung cells of white rats. When ozone gas was injected into the lungs of the rats, cell membrane lipids were peroxidized by harmful oxygen species, leading to deformation of the cell membrane and degradation of cell membrane functions. However, the authors found that when taurine was added to the cell culture medium, taurine moved into the cells so that the amount of taurine in the cells increased and toxicity was prevented.

With regard to this protective effect of taurine, Huxtable explained that taurine acts as a defense mechanism against environmental contamination or toxic substances in the living body. Therefore, for modern people exposed to pollution defenselessly, the deficiency of taurine is equivalent to the deficiency of the defense mechanism in the body that neutralizes toxicity.

## 23.7   Promotion of fat metabolism in fat tissues

Watanabe et al. (1987) gave 2 g of taurine per day for two days to nine adult males and nine adult females. The authors made the subjects run for 3 km and measured the amount of free fatty acids in the blood. In the study, adults who took taurine showed considerable increases in the amount of free fatty acids in their bodies, had better blood sugar levels, and felt less fatigue in comparison with the adults who did not take taurine. These results indicated that taurine intake during exercise induces increases in free fatty acids in the blood by promoting fat metabolism rather than saccharometabolism in the energy source supply process.

Tanaka et al. (1985) studied the effects of taurine on the supply of free fatty acids during exercise. The effect of taurine on fatty acid degradation by epinephrine was measured using epididymis fat tissues of 50-week-old white rats. Free fatty acid release from fat tissues was promoted in white rats treated with 2 to 20 μm of taurine and, in particular, the ratio of unsaturated fatty acids increased. The sympathetic nervous system is directly involved in the release of fatty acids during exercise, and catecholamine[*] promotes the degradation of fat tissues. Taurine is involved in promoting lipolysis by catecholamine, thereby promoting fat metabolism.

---

[*] *Catecholamine*: A generic term for chemicals that have an activating function and which function as neurotransmitters and hormones in the body.

## 23.8   Brain cell protection

Taurine is the most abundant component among amino acids in the vertebrate brain. In the brain, taurine shows neuromodulatory, osmoregulatory, and anticonvulsant activities. Taurine is liberated to the outsides of nerve cells during the continuous excitement of the nervous system to inhibit neuromodulatory activity and excessive excitement and exhibit nerve cell membrane protective activity and osmoregulatory functions. In addition, taurine exhibits defensive effects against nerve tissue disorders due to excitant factors. The cell membrane protection and antioxidant effects should be effective in preventing dementia by inhibiting the generation of cell membrane lipoperoxides by oxygen radicals, which are a cause of degenerative neuronal diseases.

As examined thus far, taurine acts as an important physiological functional substance in living bodies for detoxification, defense against lung damage, protection of brain cells, stimulation of fat metabolism, and control of hypertension. In addition, taurine is known to be an essential amino acid in cats, since a lack of taurine in these animals will lead to a severe weakening of the optic nerves, resulting in a reduced ability to see in the darkness. Therefore, taurine is closely associated with the normal functioning of the optic nervous system. As taurine is present in breast milk in large quantities, it is considered indispensable for the growth of newborns and the development of their nerves and brain.

# chapter twenty-four

# Antifreeze proteins in fish

## 24.1    Can frozen humans be revived?

Most human beings hope to live healthily for the natural span of their life. Although the maximum human life span is estimated to be approximately 150 years, most human beings live only half of it and die of diseases or accidents. In South Korea, at least approximately 76,000 people die of cancer per year (2014). Cancer is the largest cause of death among all diseases, and its cure rate is extremely low.

In the United States, a novel method has been developed for freezing humans suffering from incurable diseases, such as cancer, and thawing them when the medicine has been developed to revive them and treat the diseases. The method was developed in 1959 and, currently, tens of thousands of frozen human beings are sleeping at temperatures below −100°C.

When a human is frozen, a substance that prevents blood from freezing is injected into the blood, and body tissue cells may be regenerated to some extent with the aforementioned method. However, the revival of frozen humans can be regarded as impossible to date because nerve cells cannot be revived with current technology.

## 24.2    Antifreeze fish proteins

Some fish survive at temperatures of several degrees below zero. Those fish have special proteins called antifreeze proteins that prevent their body fluids from freezing in their blood or cells.

*Pagothenia borchgrevinki* does not freeze even at −19°C, which is the temperature at which sea water freezes, because it possesses antifreeze peptides in its body (Figure 24.1).

A number of antifreeze proteins in fish increase as the water temperature drops and decrease when the water temperature rises. The freezing point of the blood plasma also changes according to the amount of the antifreeze proteins present. The fluctuation in the concentration of antifreeze proteins can usually be seen only in fish that live in places in which the water temperature fluctuates according to changes in the seasons. The concentration of antifreeze proteins in the blood of fish that live in the

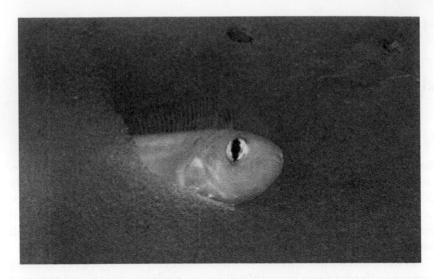

*Figure 24.1* Ice in an iceberg used as a hiding place by *Pagothenia borchgrevinki* living in the Antarctic Ocean.

Antarctic sea, where the water temperature is always below −8°C, is said to be maintained at almost constant amounts.

The antifreeze proteins discovered thus far are small proteins with molecular weights ranging from 3,000 to 30,000 kDa. Four types of proteins are known: types I, II, and III, and antifreeze proteins containing sugar.

Type I antifreeze protein is found in various species of fish inhabiting the shallow sea off the Atlantic coast of Canada in North America, contains 11 types of amino acids, and has an α helix structure rich in alanine residues, which account for 65% of the entire amino acids.

Type II antifreeze protein was discovered in fish inhabiting the reef area of the Atlantic Ocean off the coast of Canada. Its molecular weight is 14,000 kDa and it is rich in alanine (14.4%) but not as rich as type I antifreeze protein. This antifreeze protein is characterized by its cysteine-rich β structure (one of the secondary structures of proteins or polypeptides). Type III antifreeze protein was also found in fish inhabiting the water off the Atlantic coast of Canada and it is a small protein with a molecular weight of approximately 6,000 kDa. It is comprised of 15 types of amino acids, but it is different from types I or II antifreeze protein because no amino acid is present in a particularly large amount.

Those fish inhabiting the Antarctic Ocean or those inhabiting the Arctic Circle have antifreeze proteins containing sugar. These antifreeze proteins have molecular weights ranging from 2,600 to 33,000 kDa, and their primary structures are very similar and contain repeating units of alanine-alanine-threonine. Their structures are composed of disaccharides, in which threonine residues are combined with galactose and N-acetylgalactosamine.

These antifreeze proteins have shown freezing point drop effects with efficiencies of 200 to 300 times higher than those expected from the molar concentrations of the proteins present in the blood plasma. These proteins have been identified as antifreezers that drop the freezing point and bind to the surfaces of ice crystals to prevent crystal formation. Therefore, it would be possible to identify the genes of the antifreeze proteins made by fish and to mass-produce the genes through genetic engineering. Given that if the antifreeze proteins produced as such are injected in the blood of a human body before freezing, the destruction of brain cells and nerve cells may be prevented, and the human dream of reviving frozen humans may soon come true.

Medical treatment through the use of freezing methods existed in the past too. James Arnott, MD, of the United Kingdom asserted the concept of using freezing methods to inhibit tumor growth or to relieve pain in body regions that could be easily accessed by a saline solution containing ice, and freeze the cancer tissues formed in the regions using the solution. It is in this way that cryosurgery was born.

Recently, a device in which thin probes cooled by liquid nitrogen are stored was developed to reduce chill injuries. Imaging techniques such as computer tomography colonography and nuclear magnetic resonance imaging used along with the aforementioned device have greatly contributed to the advancement of cryosurgery. However, the use of these techniques has problems because they cannot be widely employed because of associated side effects caused by damage to external tissues adjacent to the affected regions resulting from the freezing. If antifreeze proteins are used, groundbreaking development of cryosurgery might be achieved.

# chapter twenty-five

# *Resolution of food shortage by fish breeding*

On October 12, 1990, Kofi Annan, the Secretary-General of the United Nations (UN), declared the birth of the world's six billionth human in a hospital in Sarajevo, Bosnia. With this revelation, it was found that the world population had increased from five to six billion in only 12 years, while in the past, the world population had taken 13 years to escalate from four to five billion—clearly showing that the rate of population growth at that point had escalated so much that it had taken one year less to increase the population count by one billion than before. It is expected that the total world population will increase from 7.32 billion in 2015 to 9.99 billion in the year 2060 (OECD Social Indicators, 2015).

One of the major issues associated with an increasing population is the production of sufficient quantities of food. Towards this end, an increase in cultivation acreage, use of chemical fertilizers and pesticides, and the cultivation of high-yield varieties are a few measures that have been implemented so as to increase the food production. However, these methods display certain limitations, such as the limited available land area that can be used for cultivation and the safety issues associated with the use of chemical fertilizers and pesticides. Therefore, plant breeding scientists have started to employ genetic engineering techniques for the efficient production of new species.

Genetic engineering has demonstrated striking development since 1953, when Watson and Crick unraveled the secret of deoxyribonucleic acid (DNA) that constitutes genes.

Recently, the swine dysentery and foot-and-mouth disease have been predominant and have resulted in the death or stamping out of numerous infected pigs. Similar to the existing human diseases, vaccines and antibiotics are the major countermeasures against diseases in domestic animals. However, the domestic animal pathogens are increasingly becoming resistant to vaccines and antibiotics, so scientists are considering other methods, such as the birth of genetically modified domestic animals that are inherently resistant to diseases. In addition, modified domestic animals that have higher growth rates or higher meat quality than current animals are also under exploration.

In early July 2015, dozens of piglets were born at the University of Edinburgh in the United Kingdom. The parents of these pigs belonged to the Yorkshire breed, which is the most commonly raised breed of the animal in the world. However, while deciphering the pig genome in 2012, the research group of the University of Edinburgh discovered a gene that reacts with pig cholera. The research team dissected the gene responsible for the pig cholera from the Yorkshire pig embryos and replaced it with a gene from warthogs, which do not contract pig cholera. Thus, the resultant progeny piglets were such that they were different from the other Yorkshire piglets only in that they possessed a pig cholera-resistant gene (Freeman et al., 2012).

## 25.1   What is marine biotechnology?

Broadly speaking, genetic engineering involves the employment of technologies as a means to use or appropriate the functions of living organisms. The core technologies of genetic engineering include gene manipulation, cell fusion, cell mass culture, and bioreactors. Genetic engineering has prompted evolution in the medical and biological fields via an immense contribution to the welfare of human beings. It is widely employed in the fields of basic studies, industries, agriculture, and animal husbandry with respect to aging, carcinogenesis and immunity, mass production of growth hormones, and pollution-free insecticides and pesticide-free agricultural products.

With the advances made in genetic engineering techniques in the area of microbiology, the scope of their application has gradually expanded to plants and animals, with wide targets, one of which is the ocean (an unexplored field by mankind), with the associated field of study being called *marine biotechnology*. Marine biotechnology is a comprehensive biotechnology area created by grafting other cutting-edge technologies on marine organisms and the ecosystems. In brief, it includes studies on cell tissue culture, cell manipulation, gene recombination, and biological engineering involving marine flora and fauna. In recent years, marine biotechnology has garnered enough limelight, especially with respect to the advent of transgenic fishes (fishes with recombinant genomes). Currently, a technology to generate only females by pressurizing the eggs to fertilize with ultraviolet-irradiated sperms has become highly usable. Such technologies that focus on the generation of females greatly aid in the aquaculture industry, such as with respect to the mass production of salmon and herring roes.

In 2012, AquaBounty Technologies, a biotechnology company in the United States, modified the salmon genes so as to produce salmons that grow at least two times faster than the typical salmon. These modified salmons possess genes from eels that render the former to grow faster and also exhibit a strong defense system against diseases. The United States Food and Drug Administration (FDA) recently permitted the aquaculture of these transgenic salmons, which are being grown in floating fish cages in Panama.

In addition, chickens that do not contract avian influenza (AI); pigs that have "omega-3," (an unsaturated fatty acid that is good for health); and cows that produce milk without the β-lactoglobulin, which is a component that causes allergy, have already been developed.

## 25.2    Future of aquatic breeding technology

Animal breeding (creating excellent breeds and improved breeds by cross-breeding) is a practice of developing animals with desired genetic traits, generally for human benefits. The breeding of farm animals for livestock products is progressing rapidly such that improved varieties of the typical dairy items become commercially available. However, the breeding of fish and shellfish, which are the targets for marine products, has been delayed, leading to the consumption of only their wild types in most cases.

In general, it is difficult to raise and breed fishes and shellfishes by the conventional measures, such as successive rearing, selection, and breeding. Moreover, there has been little interest in breeding per se, since plenty of species and large quantities are caught. However, recently, the development of efficient farming technologies has become the need of the hour due to the decreasing number of fish catches since the establishment of respective exclusive economic zones of 200 nautical miles worldwide and other problems; thus, expectations from aquaculture are increasing due to the depletion of the resources. In addition, recent years have observed a potential demand for fish and shellfish as health foods and high-grade favorite foods, and this requirement continues to grow. Towards this end, the production of groundbreaking aquaculture varieties with the traits of excellent economic value is expected.

Meanwhile, in Africa and Asia, animal protein resources are still overwhelmingly insufficient. Despite the vast inland waters and sea surfaces available in and around both continents, these resources are hardly utilized. Therefore, it is no exaggeration to say that the rapid rise in food self-sustainability depends on the development of the aquaculture of fishes and shellfishes. One of the methods to solve this problem is to develop varieties that can withstand special environmental conditions, such as water temperatures, salt concentrations, and water quality in the local areas, and that can be cultured easily.

At present, the importance of the ocean is gradually increasing in terms of a high-quality provision of protein sources and as the last food repository of mankind. Recently, a great setback in the demand and supply chain for fishery products has been expected due to the international deterioration of fishery conditions and environmental contamination factors such as coastal contamination and landfills; notably, the act of just catching fish is already unable to meet the population's demand. Moreover, the recent launch of the World Trade Organization system has marked the beginning of the era of internationalization and the opening of agricultural and marine products along with unlimited competition systems. Therefore, securing the international competitiveness of fisheries, gathering demands for the promotion of national welfare, and ensuring strategic development of technologies that can contribute to national food distribution and export strategies of fishery products by an advancement into the world market, is considered very important.

To meet such global trends and national needs, it seems imperative to maximize improved production and to increase the aquaculture yields by the development of intensive cutting-edge technologies. Among the basic requirements for aquaculture, the production of seeds (larvae) is considered the most relevant in terms of securing raw materials for the products. Furthermore, the production of good seeds is regarded as a shortcut towards maximization of the aquaculture productivity.

## 25.3   *Production of transgenic fishes*

Transgenic fishes can be produced by the cell fusion technique. Figure 25.1 demonstrates an example of the technique, wherein the cells of tropical fish, which like high water temperatures and are resistant to diseases, and salmon, which like low water temperatures and are anadromous,

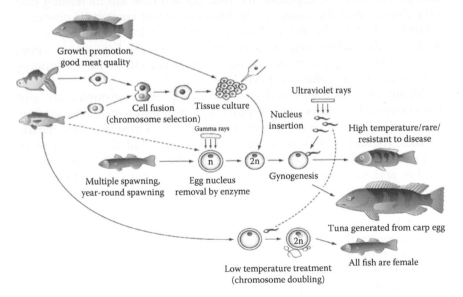

*Figure 25.1* Making transformed fish by cell fusion, nucleus transplantation, and gynogenesis.

were fused and their nuclei were transplanted into loach roes, which are easily and readily available. As a result, a transgenic progeny was produced: large fishes resistant to the diseases that are encountered while going through the warm waters of the southern sea of Japan were created. This transgenic fish displayed advantages over the other fish that like and inhabit the colder, northern sea, such as the fish that live in Russian waters.

Another example of the application of transgenic technology in marine biology is the generation of large rainbow trout by the insertion of the growth hormone gene of tuna into the genome of the former. This would result in the dramatic growth of the transgenic rainbow trout, making these animals huge and tasty like the tuna cultivated in the sea.

The extensive procedure is divided into three stages based on the regulation of the growth hormone gene to be inserted into the egg (Figure 25.2). At first, a base sequence specific to the growth hormone gene is identified to fabricate a probe of oligonucleotides (short DNA fragments with dozens of bases) that are complementary to the base sequence. To this end, the growth hormone, which is a protein molecule, is extracted from the pituitary gland (the hormone production organ) of the tuna donor and purified to analyze its amino acid sequence. The major sequences of the growth hormone gene of the tuna fish can be identified by the estimation of the corresponding DNA base sequence in the genetic code table. A specific sequence is selected from the major sequences and DNA fragments of between 20 and 50 base pairs are artificially synthesized using a DNA synthesizer.* The base sequence is then labeled with a radioactive isotope of phosphorus ($^{32}P$) to enable its function as a probe.

Following this first step, the next one is the complementary DNA (cDNA) synthesis of the growth hormone gene. The messenger ribonucleic acid (RNA; genetic information encoded by the DNA base sequence of any gene is transcribed into messenger RNA [mRNA] by RNA polymerase) is isolated from the pituitary gland, which abundantly produces and secretes growth hormones, and is subjected to synthesis of cDNA, in which the information gets replicated. The cDNA is inserted into cloning vectors (DNA vectors that can introduce desired DNA fragments into host bacteria for proliferation in recombinant DNA technique experiments), such as plasmids (closed circular DNA that exist and replicate independently of the bacterial chromosomes), and are introduced into *Escherichia coli*, cultured in large quantities, and cloned. The resulting cDNA clones constitute the cDNA library, which can be preserved and derived from various genes that were active in the pituitary gland during the extraction of the mRNA. Among the other genes, only the growth hormone cDNA fragment gets identified by the synthetic probe and cloned.

---

* *DNA Synthesizer.* A device for producing complementary DNA strands by DNA polymerase in the presence of template DNA.

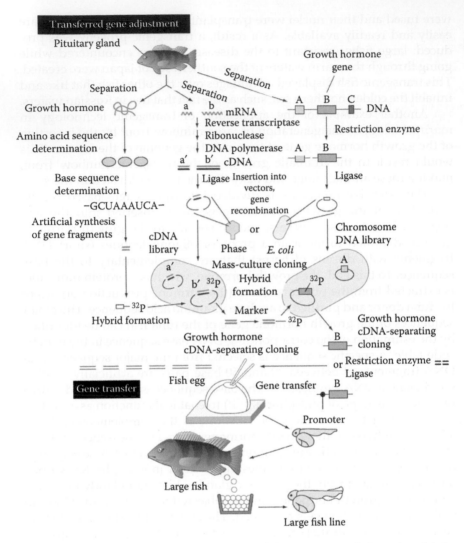

*Figure 25.2* The process by which the growth hormone gene is introduced into fish eggs.

The third step involves extraction of the growth hormone gene per se. In egg cells, rather than the cDNA without the information part, the entire gene is introduced into the cells that offer a high expression. First, the total genomic* DNA is extracted as macromolecules from the body

---

* *Genome*: The entire genetic information or the total amount of genes in a chromosome of an organism, that is, chromosomal DNA, which is the minimum gene region required to sustain life by exerting its entire functions.

tissues, such as blood cells, muscles, and so on, followed by fragmentation by restriction enzymes, ligation, and cloning in *Escherichia coli* or phages. This is called a chromosomal DNA library because it is expected to contain all of the genes on the chromosome. To select a growth hormone gene from the chromosomal DNA clones, the cDNA with a complementary sequence to the entire information portion is generally used to enable a more precise selection.

The cloned growth hormone gene is introduced into the recipient egg cell by microinjection, either as it is or in a combination with a suitable promoter gene. The steps of the introduction of the transgene into the genome of the rainbow trout (host), the expression of the transgene, and the transmission of the gene to the offspring all require stringent monitoring.

In this context, next, the kinds of genes and their resulting traits that can be introduced into fishes are considered. In the conventional breeding method (mating), the expansion of the desirable genes is limited to the organisms of the same species or those that are closely related only. However, in the gene introduction method, any gene from any species can be introduced into another species by an appropriate method. This implies that the entire gene resources, including approximately 20,000 species of fish and even those of all other living organisms currently living on the Earth (i.e., several million species), can be used.

In general, the genes that are already present in fish or similar genes are introduced to amplify the desired functions or to emphasize certain advantageous or economically valuable traits (for example, the growth hormone gene). In certain cases, entirely new genes are also introduced in different host organisms in order to allow for the expression of abilities possessed only by certain fish in other fish as well (for example, the flatfish antifreeze protein gene or carp $\alpha$-globin gene). Both of the purposes for the production of transgenic animals are important for breeding.

Since flatfish can live even in the Arctic Ocean, where the temperature is so low that it leads to the freezing of blood (though the anti-freeze protein prevents this), their gene can be introduced into salmon to expand the culture area for salmon.

While salmon and trout are vulnerable to oxygen deficiency, carp are resistant to this condition. This difference can be attributed to the dissimilar molecular structures of hemoglobin (the blood oxygen transport protein) and globin (a subunit that constitutes hemoglobin). Therefore, carp's globin gene can be introduced into rainbow trout to enhance the breathing ability of the trout so as to enable its survival in quiescent water and also its easy transportation.

Professor Kim of Pukyong National University, South Korea genetically manipulated the super loach in such a way that the transgenic fish is able to grow approximately 35 times faster than the normal loach. Moreover, a normal loach weighs only approximately 60 g even if it grows

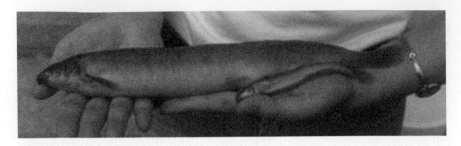

*Figure 25.3* The first super loach, developed by Professor Kim of Pukyong National University.

throughout its life span of 10 years, while the super loach can grow to weigh more than 400 g and measure up to 40 cm in length (Figure 25.3).

## 25.4 Controversy over the safety of transgenics

Genetic modifications are already common in plants and have been applied by various chemical companies, including Monsanto, DuPont, and BASF, for the development and supply of soybeans, corn, and rice that grow well in drought conditions and do not contract diseases. As of 2014, genetically modified crops have been cultivated in 13% of the total area comprised of farmland throughout the world. South Korea imported 10.82 million tons of genetically modified crops as food/raw materials and feed in the year 2014.

The most notable product of recent years is the potato, a food source that is loved all over the world. However, as the use of pesticides applied to prevent potato blight is prohibited due to the environmental contamination that results, the propagation of healthy potato crops has gradually become more difficult. To put an end to the potato's disease susceptibility, the United Kingdom and the Republic of Ireland governments are developing genetically modified potatoes, which are intended to be resistant to potato diseases and cyst nematodes.

It is expected that the farmers who continuously struggle against livestock diseases and crop blight will have little reason to dismiss the use of genetic modification technology if one huge, remaining barrier is resolved: the controversy over the safety of transgenic crops.

Although genetic modification has been applied to plants for more than two decades now, the side effects that may appear upon consumption of genetically modified crops by humans have not been thoroughly elucidated. Furthermore, though some scientists have a collective opinion that genetically modified crops should now be regarded as being safe, since their harmfulness has not been proven, such comments seem to be insufficient to persuade the general public.

At present, consumers are demanding a qualitative improvement in the cultured fish that can be stably produced at a mass-scale, in the hope that they will be able to see the fish on the table as a safer and tastier food item. The desired qualitative improvement can be achieved by *breeding (breed improvement)*, which only becomes possible with the understanding of the *genetic traits*.

Recently, in addition to the genetic manipulation of organisms to enable the production of useful substances for mass production or treatment, the use of methods to maximally utilize the inheritability of living organisms, such as selective breeding based on gene markers, have also been attempted.

Notably, it is believed that fish species that are resistant to diseases and are highly adaptive to temperature changes can reduce the occurrence of fish diseases so that they can be cultivated without supplementation of medicines or antibiotics, subsequently fulfilling consumers' demands for safe food. In addition, fish with good meat quality can meet consumer choice, and fish with high growth potential can reduce production costs, thus also satisfying customers due to the low production costs and thus reduced market prices.

# chapter twenty-six

# Development of functional cosmetic materials from marine organisms

In South Korea, diverse traditional therapies and folk remedies, known as East Asian medicine, have been in practice for many years. Most of these use terrestrial plants as their ingredients, but there are some that also use components derived from the ocean. This also applies to the products in the cosmetic industry that are created based on the raw materials used in the traditional means of therapy. Meanwhile, in Europe, there are various traditional therapies using components obtained from the ocean such as seaweed, seawater, and sea mud, which are also called *thalassotherapy*.

Recently, thalassotherapy has been introduced to South Korea, and the interest in marine products has been increasing, especially among females. In addition, due to the problems of bovine spongiform encephalopathy (BSE), there has been a common tendency to avoid raw materials obtained from terrestrial mammals, and consequently, interest in marine living organisms as an alternative source of raw materials has rapidly increased.

Cosmetics are the substances applied in several ways to clean or embellish the body, increase attractiveness, change the actual looks, or keep the hair soft, which have mild to moderate actions on the human body. Hence, cosmetics have mild effects aimed at improving skin or hair conditions through long-term usage and do not pose strong effects, unlike medicines. In addition to having only mild effects, the raw materials should be suitable for cosmetic products, skin friendly, and should have a good identity.

Marine algae are regarded as an excellent source of raw ingredients for the cosmetic industry, since they comply with all of the above-mentioned criteria. The details of all of the raw materials approved for use in various cosmetic preparations have been thoroughly discussed in official compendium of relevant knowledge that includes the *Cosmetic Raw Material Standard* and *Standards for Mix Components by Type of Cosmetics*.

Since the regulations on cosmetic products have been relaxed at present; the cosmetic raw materials need not to be necessarily listed in the aforementioned official compendium. However, the standards listed in the official compendium are very useful criteria for ascertaining the safety and quality of these products.

The details of marine products reproduced from the official compendium are summarized in Table 26.1. The cosmetics that contain skin-friendly biomolecules extracted from natural substances or bioprocessed to strengthen skin anti-aging and whitening properties are called *functional bio-cosmetics*. Since the bioactive ingredients are added to these cosmetic products to have beauty treatment effects, they are also called *cosmeceuticals*, a term derived from the combination of *cosmetics* and *pharmaceuticals*.

There are seven major functions of cosmetics: skin moisturizing, anti-oxidation, protection against ultraviolet (UV) rays, wrinkle improvement,

*Table 26.1*  Marine-derived cosmetic raw materials in the pharmacopoeia-approved precedents

| Name | Raw material | Name | Raw material |
|------|-------------|------|-------------|
| Potassium alginate | Brown algae | Agar powder | Agar |
| Sodium alginate | Brown algae | Desulfurized aluminum silicate | Sea mud |
| Calcium alginate | Brown algae | Chitin | Snow crab and red snow crab |
| Sodium propylene glycol alginate | Brown algae | Chitosan | Crustaceans |
| Sodium sulfate alginate | Brown algae | Fish scale | Largehead hairtail |
| Squid ink | Squid | Chlorella extract | Chlorella |
| *Laticauda semifasciata* lipid | *Laticauda semifasciata* | Succinyl chitosan | Crustaceans |
| Sea water dry matter | Sea water | Squalene | Shark |
| Seaweed extract | Brown, red and green algae | Squalane | Deep sea sharks |
| Hydrolysate extract | Squid | Water-soluble collagen | Fish |
| Oyster extract | Oyster | Conchiolin powder | Pearl oyster |
| Carrageenan | Red algae | Pearl powder | Shellfish |
| Carboxymethyl chitin solution | Crabs | Hydroxyethyl chitosan solution | Crustaceans |
| Dried chlorella | Chlorella | Hydroxypropyl chitosan solution | Crustaceans |

skin tone whitening, the prevention of acne, hair growth, and aromatic effects. Recently, edible cosmetics (*nutricosmetics*) have also emerged to delineate the boundary between cosmetics and foods. Thus, due to the advent of modern technologies such as gene manipulation and bioprocess engineering and the introduction of useful natural resource search tools, bio-cosmetics are expanding exponentially to the field of pharmaceuticals and dietetics.

In the last decade, it was investigated for the inclusion of marine ingredients such as seaweeds and seawater dry matter, and a rapid upsurge was noticed with respect to the utilization of marine components as cosmetics since the 2000s. Thereafter, it can be said that at this time, the trend of avoiding raw materials derived from mammals and birds began to increase, and marine products started attracting attention as a novel source. Among the various kinds of marine products used in cosmetic formulations, marine algae are the most frequently used example, followed by sea salt and sea mud, in order of prevalence.

The different actions of marine raw materials on the skin are mentioned in Table 26.2. The scope of application of polysaccharides extracted from seaweeds such as agar, alginic acid, and carrageenan has been rapidly growing, owing to their properties. Among them, alginic acid, a polymer of D-mannuronic acid and L-gluronic acid, shows high viscosity and is obtained from brown algae such as kelp, sea mustard, *Sargassum horneri*, and seaweed *Fusiforme*. It is currently being used as a natural thickener in cosmetics. Carrageenan, an acidic polysaccharide composed of galactose and anhydrogalactose, is also used as a stabilizer or dispersant in cosmetics.

*Table 26.2* Effects of marine compounds as per the published patents

| | |
|---|---|
| Seaweeds | *Skin care cosmetics*: Moisturizing, skin chapping prevention, promotion of hyaluronic acid production, promotion of collagen production, fibroblast-promoting effect, elastinase inhibition, antioxidation |
| Sea water and sea salt | *Bath preparation*: Skin moisturizing, skin chapping prevention and improvement<br>*Skin care cosmetic*: Whitening effect, skin moisturizing, skin chapping prevention |
| Sea mud | *Detergents*: Scrub effect<br>*Pack*: Moisturizing effect, skin waste removal effect, etc.<br>*Skin care cosmetics*: Moisturizing effect, whitening effect<br>*Hair care cosmetics*: To gain a feeling of smoothness, moisturizing property |

## 26.1    The Sun as a concern

The planet Earth where we live is an integral part of the solar system and no living thing on Earth can survive without the Sun. Although sunlight is a prime source of energy and indispensable for the survival of mankind, its UV radiation causes serious harm to humans. Recently, environmental pollution has become a serious threat due to the Industrial Revolution. Consequently, the ozone layer in the atmosphere has depleted, leading to a rapid increase in the amount of UV rays reaching the surface of the Earth.

Furthermore, due to modernization and cultural shifts, the chance of UV-ray exposure is also increasing. As the participation in leisure and sport activities is rising, the higher frequency of traveling to regions in the vicinity of the Equator characterized by an extremely high UV index is leading to a growing interest in understanding the effects of UV rays on the human body and in methods to protect the skin by blocking these UV rays.

### 26.1.1    What are UV rays?

The sunlight regime consists of gamma rays, X-rays, UV rays, visible rays, infrared rays, and radio waves. Visible rays are a colored light spectrum that can be seen with the eyes. UV rays are of a shorter wavelength than the violet rays of the visible spectrum. UV rays are divided into UV A (320–400 nm), UV B (280–320 nm), and UV C (200 ~ 280 nm) with long, medium, and short wavelengths, respectively.

UV A light rays with long wavelengths are weak in energy but pass through glass and penetrate the epidermal layer of the skin to convert the light-color melanin pigment into dark color, leading to tanning. It also deforms collagen and elastin to reduce elasticity, thereby causing skin wrinkles and aging, and is involved in the onset of photosensitive skin diseases. Unlike UV B, most of the UV A rays pass through fog and window glass and most reach the ground even on cloudy days.

Whereas most of the UV B rays are absorbed by the epidermis, UV A rays penetrate deep into the epidermis and prolonged exposure possibly leads to the loss of skin elasticity. UV B rays are high-energy light rays with short wavelengths that penetrate the epidermis in a short time to cause skin erythema, sunburn (a phenomenon that burns the skin to turn it reddish), blisters, and rash, and increases melanin pigment in a few days to cause *hyperpigmentation* (suntan) on the skin (Figure 26.1).

### 26.1.2    UV rays and ozone

The ozone layer in the stratosphere, located approximately 13 to 50 km above the Earth's surface, plays the role of a protective film that shields

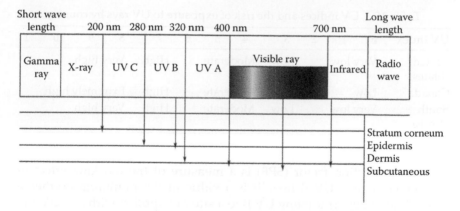

*Figure 26.1* Sunlight ranges and dermal penetration.

humans and other living things from the hazardous UV rays of the Sun. Unfortunately, in the early 1980s, scientists began to notice the destruction of the stratospheric ozone layer.

As the degree of environmental air pollution progressed seriously with industrial development, the ozone layer also started depleting such that it fails to block UV rays, which eventually led to an increase in the amount of UV B rays reaching the Earth's surface. This phenomenon results in skin hyperpigmentation, cataract, skin wrinkle formation, and skin aging, and has various adverse effects on human health such as skin cancer and the loss of the immune system efficacy.

An oxygen molecule ($O_2$) in the atmosphere is dissociated into two oxygen atoms (O) by UV rays, and the oxygen atoms combine with another oxygen molecule ($O_2$) to form ozone ($O_3$). The layer formed by the ozone molecules collectively is called the ozone layer. In this way, the UV rays of the Sun naturally maintain the balance of the ozone layer in the stratosphere and the ozone protects living organisms on the Earth from UV rays.

## 26.1.3   What is the UV Index?

The UV Index provides a forecast of the expected risks due to overexposure to the Sun's rays, thereby presenting the degree to which we should be careful with respect to UV rays in our daily lives. The UV Index is divided into a scale of 10 grades, where 0 indicates that the risk expected due to an overexposure is very low and 9 indicates that the risk expected is very high. There may be some differences in the way to distinguish the indices in different countries (Table 26.3).

*Table 26.3* UV indices and the risk of exposure to UV rays by country

| UV index | 0 | 1 | 2 | 3 | 4 | 5 | 6 | 7 | 8 | 9 | 10 | 11 |
|---|---|---|---|---|---|---|---|---|---|---|---|---|
| United States | Very low | | | Low | Moderate | | | High | Very high | | | |
| Canada | Low | | | | Moderate | | | High | Extremely high | | | |
| South Korea | Very low | | | Low | Moderate | | | High | Very high | | | |

Sun protection factor (SPF) is a measure of the blocking effect of a product against UV B rays. It is a value of the minimum erythema dose obtained by irradiating UV B to a site not applied with any UV-ray blocking product divided by the minimum erythema dose obtained by irradiating UV B to a site applied with the UV-ray blocking product.

The SPF is a value that indicates the degree to which sunburn is prevented and how long the skin can be exposed to the sun without burning. For example, if the SPF is assumed to be 15 (SPF 15) and the mean MED for South Koreans is assumed to be 37 $mJ/cm^3$, the maximum amount of the light to which the skin can be exposed will be 555 $mJ/cm^3$ (maximum quantity of light = 37 $mJ/cm^3 \times 15 = 555$ $mJ/cm^3$). Therefore, if the quantity of light is 370 $mJ/cm^3$, the skin can be exposed for one hour and 30 minutes ($555/370 = 1.5$ h) and, if the quantity of light is 550 $mJ/cm^3$.day, then the skin can be exposed for one day. However, products with higher SPF should be used for weaker and more sensitive skins, as the mean MED values are lower for such skins (Table 26.4).

In addition, the time that is taken for the first incidence of erythema to occur when the bare skin is exposed to sunlight also varies among different human races. It is approximately 15 minutes in Caucasians, 20 minutes in Mongoloids, and 25 minutes in Negroids. Therefore, when SPF 20 products are used, ultraviolet rays can be blocked for 300 minutes in case of Caucasians (SPF 20 $\times$ 15 min = 300 min), 400 minutes in Mongoloids (SPF 20 $\times$ 20 min = 400 min), and 500 minutes in Negroids (SPF 20 $\times$ 25 min = 500 min).

*Table 26.4* Comparison of SPF according to UV indices

| UV index | 0 | 1 | 2 | 3 | 4 | 5 | 6 | 7 | 8 | 9 | 10 | 11 |
|---|---|---|---|---|---|---|---|---|---|---|---|---|
| Quantity of light[a] | 0 | 50 | 100 | 150 | 200 | 250 | 300 | 350 | 400 | 450 | 500 | 550 |
| Risk of exposure | Very low | | | Low | | Moderate | | High | | Very high | | |
| SPF | <4 | | | 4–7 | | 7–9 | | 9–12 | | 12–15 | | |

[a] Unit of the quantity of light: $mJ/cm^2$-day; Minimal erythema dose (MED): 37 $mJ/cm^2$.

However, the duration of the blocking efficacy can further vary depending upon environmental or physical conditions such as sweating or due to the very high intensity of UV rays.

## 26.1.4 Sunscreen agents

The UV-ray absorbents and the UV-ray scattering agents are collectively called *sunscreen agents*. These sunscreen agents are blended in an appropriate proportion to manufacture UV-ray blocking cosmetics. Recently, a technology has been developed to make a highly water-resistant thin coating on the skin surface, which prevents makeup from being scattered and protects the skin by blocking UV rays.

### 26.1.4.1 UV-ray absorbents

These compounds absorb UV rays of between 280 and 400 nm wavelengths to protect the skin from damage. Usually, the thermal energy of UV rays absorbed by organic compounds is transformed into another form of energy before release. Therefore, the UV-ray absorbents used in cosmetics do not cause damage and are safe. These UV-ray absorbents are wavelength-specific and most of them absorb UV B. Currently, only a few absorb UV A.

### 26.1.4.2 UV-ray scattering agents

Inorganic powders, especially titanium oxide and zinc oxide, physically scatter UV rays. These powders look white as they scatter the visible UV rays. Therefore, they are used as a white color pigment in foundations and emulsion type cosmetics. However, due to their relatively larger particle sizes (0.5 µm), the scattering effect of the powders on UV rays was inadequate. Therefore, particles of approximately 0.02 µm in size were developed with two times the refractive indices so as to increase the scattering effect. In addition, the higher degree of atomization facilitated the high content mixing into lotions or creams and led to an even whitening effect without any visibility on the skin.

Titanium oxide and zinc oxide are more commonly used as UV A-blocking agents rather than as scattering agents, due to their higher blocking efficacy and, in comparison with UV-ray absorbents, a lower selectivity depending on their scattering wavelengths. In recent years, advanced technologies have been developed to block UV rays of different wavelengths by adjusting particle sizes and dispersing the particulate powder in emulsions.

### 26.1.4.3 Development of sunscreen agents from marine algae

At Jeju National University, Professor Jeon and his team conducted clinical tests on the experimental animal model system and showed that dieckol, a polyphenol extracted from marine algae, blocks UV rays more efficiently.

As apparent from Figure 26.2a, the lymphocytes of blood were changed from their normal spherical shapes to long-tailed cells by the UV exposure. However, when the cells were treated with dieckol prior to UV irradiation, the damage was more minor, indicating that dieckol blocked the UV rays and protected the cells. When animal experiments were conducted with rats, as shown in Figure 26.2b, the regions applied with dieckol did not show erythema or edema after UV irradiation, unlike the regions that were not treated with dieckol (control), demonstrating the excellent UV-ray blocking activity of the marine algae extract.

In fact, when UV-blocking test products were made and primary human skin irritation experiments were conducted at concentrations of 0.5% to 1%, which was about 100 to 1,000 times higher than the typical concentrations applied in cosmetics, stimulation within the minimum range was shown.

No other sense of subjective irritation such as stinging or itching was found with the stimulation. This confirms that dieckol can be used as a very effective and safe ingredient in UV-ray blocking products, which do not cause skin irritation.

There are sometimes complaints of side effects associated with conventional sunscreen agents because they are chemically synthesized and meant to block only UV rays. The sunscreen agent made of dieckol extracted from algae is a new type of sunscreen, which is skin-friendly and provides diverse functions ranging from whitening to anti-aging. Therefore, the use of dieckol has the potential to promote the development of the functional cosmetics industry and to strengthen the competitiveness of the currently existing functional cosmetics.

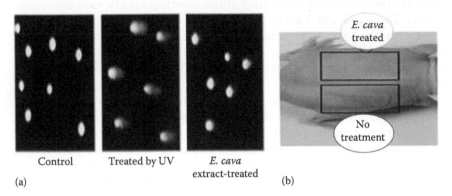

(a)          Control          Treated by UV          *E. cava*
                                                   extract-treated          (b)

*Figure 26.2* Cell protection effects of dieckol in lymphocytes as shown by UV-ray exposure (a) and the UV-ray blocking effects of dieckol in rats as an animal model (b).

## 26.2 Wrinkle improvement

Wrinkles are generally classified into fine wrinkles and large wrinkles. Fine wrinkles, which are also called epidermal wrinkles, are caused by the drying of the epidermis. Therefore, these wrinkles are more closely related with moisturizing and barrier improvement, while the large wrinkles that appear on the eye rims, around the mouth, and on the face are formed due to quantitative and qualitative changes in the epidermal matrix and the basement membrane.

The major dermal cell membrane matrixes are collagen fibers, elastin (strong fiber), and glycosaminoglycan (GAG).

When the skin is exposed to light, collagen, which accounts for the majority of the dermal matrixes, is markedly decreased and the fiber bundles are reported to be scattered. In this regard, an increase in the amount of dermal collagen is thought to be useful for wrinkle improvement or defense. Collagen is produced by dermal fibroblasts, but it is well known that collagen synthesis by fibroblasts is greatly reduced by the sub-lethal dose of UVt rays (UV B) with small amounts of energy.

Fibroblast-derived matrix metalloproteinase-1 (MMP-1) and neutrophil-derived serine protease are the enzymes that mediate the collagen degradation.

When fibroblasts are exposed to UV rays, the synthesis of MMP-1 is accelerated, leading to an increase in the neutrophil-derived collagen degradation enzyme at the inflammation site. Inhibiting the action of the collagen degradation enzyme may be an effective approach to suppress the degradation of dermal collagen.

In the regions not exposed to light, elastin increases slightly and causes thickening due to aging, but no remarkable changes are recognized; however, on the light exposure, the elastin fibers of the skin increase substantially and lead to the thickening of fibers, eventually forming amorphous masses. Elastin in its denatured form cannot function normally. Therefore, inhibiting the quantitative and qualitative changes in elastin could be useful for improving or delaying wrinkles.

When the skin is inflamed by UV rays, vascular endothelial growth factor (VEGF) production is accelerated while the amount of inhibitory factor thrombospondin-1 (TSP-1, multifunctional glycoprotein released from platelet α granules) is reduced. As a result, angiogenesis is induced so that elastin fibers are degraded by the elastase derived from serine protease and infiltrated into the regions around the blood vessels. Other elastin degradation enzymes include metal protease. Inhibiting the activity of these enzymes could effectively inhibit the quantitative and qualitative changes in elastin.

## 26.2.1  Changes in the basement membrane

The basement membrane binds to the epidermis and dermis strongly by its structure, gives mechanical strength to the skin, and regulates the communication between the dermis and the epidermis by fluidic factors. However, aging or UV exposure accelerates the degradation of laminin (a major glycoprotein that constitutes the basement membrane) and type IV collagen by gelatinases such as MMP-2 and MMP-9, or by plasmin (an enzyme that catalyzes the hydrolysis of the skin dermis), leading to a faster rate of damage to the basement membrane and, hence, photoaging occurs. Therefore, the compounds that promote the synthesis of basement membrane ingredients or inhibitors of gelatinase and plasminogen activators can be efficient inhibitors of basement membrane damage.

## 26.2.2  Active oxygen as a cause of wrinkles

The onset of cellular oxidative stress due to UV rays has been known to cause wrinkles. When human dermal fibroblasts are irradiated with UV rays (UV B), collagen synthesis is significantly reduced. Reactive oxygen species (ROS; $\bullet O^{2-}$, $H_2O_2$, $\bullet OH$) produced by xanthine-xanthine oxidase inhibit collagen synthesis.

When human fibroblasts are irradiated with UV rays (UV B), the synthesis of elastin is accelerated. However, the accumulated elastin cannot function normally as resilient fibers resisting the degradation enzyme because it is cross-linked and denatured.

The mode of action of UV rays and ROS in the dermal matrix decomposition system is described in the ensuing text.

When fibroblasts are irradiated with UV rays (UV A), the MMP-1 gene (messenger ribonucleic acid; mRNA), which is involved in the formation of wrinkles, is overexpressed. This is due to the singlet oxygen produced by UV rays. In addition, the expression of the MMP-2 gene (mRNA) in epidermal cells increases due to the exposure to the xanthine-xanthine oxidase system.

MMP synthesized as a precursor is secreted to the extracellular spaces and then converted into an active form through proteolysis by other proteases. Therefore, multiple MMPs produced by various ROS undergo cleanup processes, leading to qualitative and quantitative changes in the dermal matrix.

Although the human body produces various antioxidative factors (glutathione, which increases the cell metabolism and oxygen use efficiency of the skin, and peroxidase, super oxide dismutase (SOD), catalase, and enzymes that catalyze the reactions that decompose hydrogen peroxide) to scavenge these ROS, the antioxidative factors decrease with aging. For example, the skin loses flexibility and develops wrinkles due to changes in the dermal matrix component synthesis/decomposition systems.

### 26.2.3   Wrinkle improvement effects of MMP-1 inhibition by chitosan oligosaccharides

The effect of chitosan oligosaccharides of different molecular weights was investigated on the activity (Figure 26.3) and expression (Figure 26.4) of MMP-1 using human skin cells, and it was reported that chitosan oligosaccharides of 3 to 5 kDa molecular weight inhibited the expression.

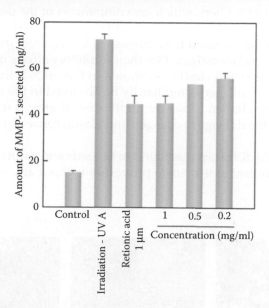

*Figure 26.3* Collagenase MMP-1 activity-suppressing effects of chitosan oligosaccharide by UV A irradiation.

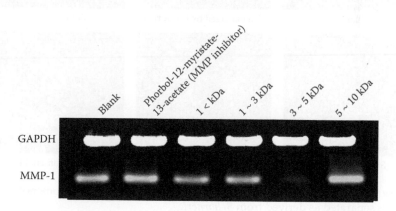

*Figure 26.4* Effects of different molecular weight chitosan oligosaccharide to inhibit the expression of MMP-1 in fibroblasts.

Since chitosan oligosaccharides can prevent wrinkle formation by inhibiting the expression of MMP, they can potentially be explored as an ingredient of functional cosmetics.

### 26.2.4 Development of wrinkle improvers from Sargassum horneri

Collagen and elastin fibers, which are components of the dermis, may be degraded by UV rays to cause skin wrinkles and reduce elasticity.

The compounds isolated from *Sargassum horneri* were irradiated with UV rays (UV A) and investigated for their inhibitory effects on the decomposition of collagen and elastin. As shown in Figure 26.5, the presence of green-fluorescent collagen could hardly be observed in the control group following UV irradiation. However, in the case of groups treated with *S. horneri* extract, the damage to collagen and elastin caused by UV rays was minimal.

The extract of *S. horneri* was found to be a safe and natural marine substance with excellent anti-wrinkle properties without any side effects on

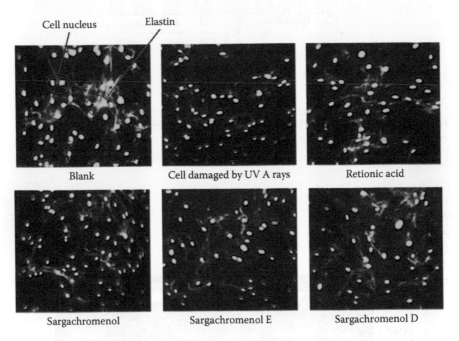

**Figure 26.5** Elastin decomposition inhibitory effect of sargachromenol compounds separated as derived from *S. horneri*.

the skin. This has not been used previously and therefore has enormous potential to be employed as a multifunctional cosmetic ingredient.

## 26.3 Whitening cosmetics

Recently, as the average life span of humans has extended, anti-aging products have been increasingly flooding the market, and cosmetics aimed at preventing and/or managing the signs of aging are no more a rare exception. Among cosmetics, whitening products are significantly popular, as they keep the face beautiful at all times. These whitening cosmetics are being developed using research on the mechanism of melanin production that causes hyperpigmentation such as melasma and freckles or sunburn.

In cosmetics, the term *whitening* refers to the maintenance of the original color of the face, rather than making the face look whiter.

Whitening cosmetics show whitening effects and restore the original tone of the skin by preventing or removing freckles or pigmentation that may present due to aging, and so on. Therefore, in order to develop whitening agents, the mechanism of the development of pigmentation should be well-understood. Novel whitening agents can only be developed after subjecting them to thorough whitening evaluation tests based on the onset mechanism.

### 26.3.1 Why does pigmentation occur?

One of the worries that can arise after a summer vacation is whether the skin has turned dark. Once the face, the back of the neck, arms, and other areas turn dark after exposure to sunlight, it takes quite a long amount of time to restore these areas to their original states. In light of this, one might ask, *why does the skin turn black when it receives sunlight?* The main cause of dark skin colors in the summer is UV rays. In order of from the most superficial layer of the epidermis to the deepest, there are five skin layers: the stratum corneum, stratum lucidum, granular layer, papillary layer, and basal layer. When UV rays stimulate the skin basal layer, the amino acid tyrosine is oxidized. The oxidized tyrosine serves as a fuel for making melanocytes that produce melanin pigment. As the amount of the fuel increases, large volumes of melanin are produced.

Melanin synthesis in the melanocytes present in the skin, hair, eyes, and so on is stimulated by UV rays or hormones. Melanin is a dark brown-colored pigment; thus, a larger amount of melanin pigment makes the skin appear darker. In this regard, the reason for skin color variations

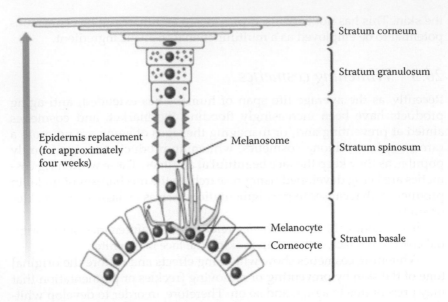

*Figure 26.6* Cross-sectional diagram of human dermis.

among the races is the size of the melanocytes and the amount of melanin pigment produced by them (Figure 26.6).

The melanin pigment in the basal layer gradually rises toward the stratum corneum over a period of time. It takes quite some time for the melanin to completely reach up to the stratum corneum. This is the reason why the skin looks darker after prolonged exposure to sunlight.

In fact, melanin pigment is not harmful to the human body; rather, it plays a role in preventing UV rays from penetrating deep into the dermal layer that eventually may cause cancer, freckles, wrinkles, and so on. Excessive exposure to UV rays should be avoided as it may cause skin problems due to the UV-ray blocking limitations of melanin pigment.

For skin that has been darkened to recover its original state, the basal layer cells that have not been stimulated by UV rays must again rise to the stratum corneum. However, when persistent intense UV rays are received, the melanin pigment may spread to the entire epidermal layer and the skin color would turn semi-permanently dark (Figure 26.7).

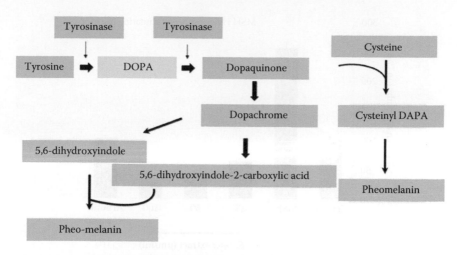

*Figure 26.7* Melanin biosynthetic pathway.

## 26.3.2 Development of whitening cosmetics from marine algae

More than 20 types of marine algal extracts were assessed for their skin-whitening properties. Among them, the activity of marine algae extract was significantly higher than that of arbutin. Active compounds were evaluated and 7-phloroeckol present in the extract was found to be a strong inhibitor of melanin synthesis (Figure 26.8).

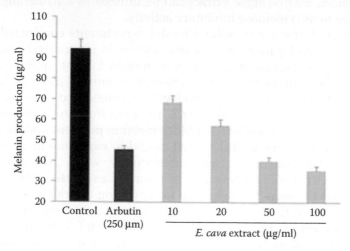

*Figure 26.8* Effects of *Ecklonia cava* extract to inhibit melanin production.

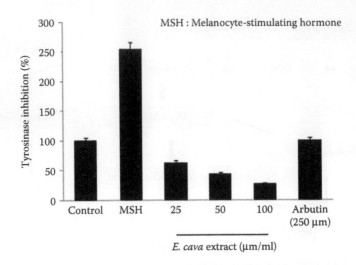

*Figure 26.9* Effects of marine algae extract to inhibit tyrosinase production.

In addition, the activity of various algal extracts against tyrosinase, an important enzyme for skin whitening, was estimated, and the marine algae extract showed approximately 50% tyrosinase inhibitory activity at a concentration of 100 ug/mL, which is higher than that of the positive control arbutin (40%) (Figure 26.9).

Therefore, marine algae extract can be utilized as a whitening compound due to its tyrosinase inhibitory activity.

At present, the use of animal model experiments conducted with rats for the development of cosmetic materials is strictly being regulated by experimental ethical laws mainly in Europe, and therefore there is an urgent need for new alternative animal models. In this regard, zebrafish as a model system has been considered to be very useful for cosmetics-related studies. As is apparent from the name, zebrafish contain very large amounts of black melanin pigment and therefore can be used as a very useful animal model in experiments related to examining the whitening effect. Interestingly, when zebrafish were irradiated with UV B rays, melanin pigment expressed abundantly, which shows the model's usefulness for verifying UV-ray blocking efficacy. In Figure 26.10, the control group zebrafish A(i) shows the normal amount of melanin, but when it is irradiated with UV B (50 mJ/cm$^2$), the expression of melanin rises very high. When it was treated with polyphenolic compounds derived from marine algae, it showed a significant reduction in melanin content. Therefore, it was concluded that the marine algae extract clearly blocks UV rays and inhibits melanin pigmentation in the skin.

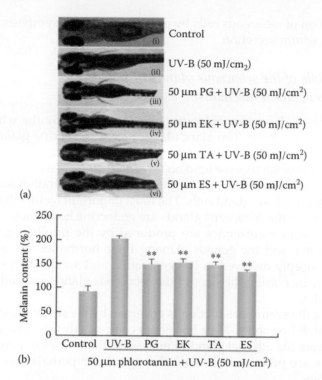

Control

UV-B (50 mJ/cm$_2$)

50 μm PG + UV-B (50 mJ/cm$^2$)

50 μm EK + UV-B (50 mJ/cm$^2$)

50 μm TA + UV-B (50 mJ/cm$^2$)

50 μm ES + UV-B (50 mJ/cm$^2$)

(a)

(b) 50 μm phlorotannin + UV-B (50 mJ/cm$^2$)

*Figure 26.10* Melanin pigment reducing the activity of marine algae resulting from UV-ray blocking in a zebrafish animal model treated with UV rays to induce melanin pigment. (a) The melanin pigment appeared in the zebrafish and (b) the increase in melanin pigment in the zebrafish.

## 26.4 Sebum control cosmetics

The functions of sebaceous glands* are regulated by multiple hormones. Androgen, a male hormone, is most closely involved in sebum production. The androgens are produced in the testes or ovaries and reach the target tissues through the blood, and testosterone, secreted from the testicles, is the most important androgen.

The expression of androgen in the target tissues requires 5α-reductase enzyme. This enzyme converts androgen into a more active male hormone known as dihydrotestosterone (DHT). This DHT or testosterone binds to and activates the androgen receptor present in sebaceous glandular cells. This activated receptor acts as a transcription enhancer to facilitate the

---

* *Sebaceous gland*: Hypodermal glands of the skin and all oil glands connected to the pores that secrete and discharge on an average between 1 and 2 g of sebum per day on the skin surface.

multiplication of sebaceous cells by promoting mRNA synthesis, thereby increasing sebum secretion.

### 26.4.1    Role of the sebaceous glands in the sebum generation mechanism

The sebaceous glands are holocrine glands that destroy the whole cells and release the sebum. The glandulae sebaceae (holocrine glands in the skin that secrete sebum) contain fat droplets as they are differentiated and finally burst to discharge the lipid on the skin surface as sebum. Therefore, the amount of sebum depends on the degree of proliferation and differentiation of sebaceous gland cells. The most important factors that control the functions of the sebaceous glands are endocrine hormones.

The endocrine hormones are produced by the pituitary gland, the adrenal cortex, and the gonads. Among these hormones, the male hormones are deeply involved in the generation and acceleration of sebum secretion by increasing the sizes of the sebaceous glands and cell division (Figure 26.11).

Most of the sebum production is governed by the sex hormones, especially the male hormones. Male hormones come mostly from the testes and partially from the adrenal gland in males and the ovaries in females, and all of these are produced/secreted through the hypothalamus-pituitary gland system.

As mentioned earlier, testosterone is metabolized into 5α-DHT by the 5α-reducing enzyme present in the sebaceous glands, and the 5α-DHT binds to the male hormone receptors of sebaceous glands to enhance the biosynthesis of lipid. Excessively produced sebum causes various

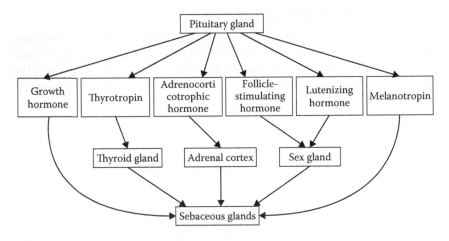

*Figure 26.11* Hormones that affect the sebaceous glands.

problems such as acne, inflammation, and collapse of the cysts. Therefore, the sebaceous gland cells of humans and hamsters can be explored to investigate the factors that control the functions of the sebaceous glands and subsequently for the development of new sebum-preventing and sebum-improving products in skin care.

### 26.4.2   Development of sebum control cosmetics from extracts of glasswort, a halophyte

Sebum is skin waste that is secreted from the pores of the skin. The excessive secretion of sebum can cause acne and skin inflammation. Recently, responses from consumers have positively increased toward cosmetics made from natural ingredients, which overwhelmingly necessitates the development of functional compounds derived from living marine organisms.

An extract from glasswort was prepared using fermented spirits, which is harmless to the human body. Thereafter, active compounds were isolated from the extract. After inducing neutral fat synthesis by treating the cells with linoleic acid, the level of efficacy of the glasswort extract was evaluated for the inhibition of neutral fat accumulation in sebocytes in a dose-dependent manner (Figure 26.12).

In addition, when human sebocytes were co-treated with linoleic acid and *Smilax herbacea* extract for 24 hours, the glasswort extract inhibited fat accumulation in sebocytes. Peroxisome proliferator-activated receptor-α

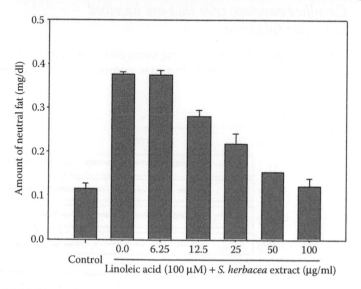

*Figure 26.12* Neutral fat production inhibitory effects of linoleic acid and *S. herbacea* extract.

(PPARα) and peroxisome proliferator-activated receptor-γ (PPARγ) hormone receptors are present in the cell nuclei and act as transcription factors that regulate lipid metabolism and sterol regulatory element-binding protein-1 (SREBP-1) and protein-β (CCAAT/enhancer-binding protein beta; C/EBPβ), which in turn promotes antioxidative functions involved in the accumulation of lipids. All of these factors are related with lipogenesis, and their reduced expression inhibits the lipogenesis.

The effect of glasswort extract was examined on the expression levels of these factors and the expression of these factors was found to be inhibited in a dose-dependent manner; in particular, there was a remarkable reduction in the expression levels at high concentrations (100 µg/mL) (Figure 26.13).

Therefore, it is proposed that glasswort extract inhibits the expression of these factors and consequently inhibits fat production in sebocytes.

In clinical tests, the effects of glasswort extract on sebum control, oil contents in the glabella, and the tip of the nose, where the sebum secretion is the most active, were quantitated and the results indicated a noticeable reduction in the oil content of the skin surface in both regions after using the sample for one to two weeks (Figure 26.14).

In conclusion, the glasswort extract inhibited the expression of fat-producing genes in sebocytes; this advocates that it can be used as a sebum-improving cosmetic ingredient due to its anti-fat activity in clinical tests.

### 26.4.3 Cornified envelope cells that are involved in barrier functions

Although the cornified envelope has long been considered useless as dead skin cells, recently, not only experts but also common users of cosmetics

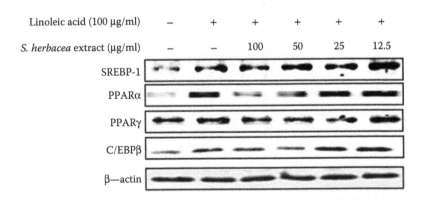

*Figure 26.13* Effects of glasswort extract to reduce intracellular fat production.

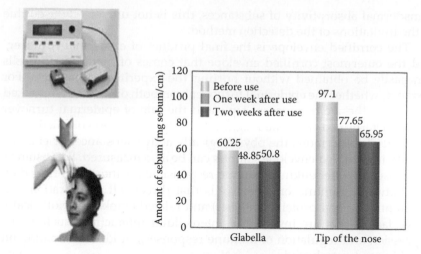

*Figure 26.14* Sebum secretion inhibitory effect of glasswort extract (clinical test results).

have come to recognize that the cornified envelope that is present in the skin plays important roles until it sheds as dead skin cells.

The skin as an outermost covering serves as an interface between the body and its surroundings. Although the cornified envelope is thin, measuring only approximately 20 μm in thickness, it protects the living body from a variety of external stimuli and prevents water evaporation from the skin: while acting as a barrier, it maintains the water content in the body amounting to about 70% and prevents the invasion of microorganisms or foreign substances such as chemicals.

However, when the cornified envelope is poorly formed, the barring and the moisture-retaining function of the skin are reduced, leading to symptoms such as dryness, desquamation (a phenomenon in which the skin epidermis comes off as fragments of the stratum corneum), and dandruff. A well-developed normal cornfield envelope helps to maintain smooth, moist, beautiful, and healthy skin. Therefore, the evaluation of the cornified envelope is considered to be an important method in determining the dryness and barrier properties of the skin.

Intensive studies are underway to develop technologies for quantitative analysis of the natural moisturizing factors (NMF; water-soluble amino acids) in keratinocytes and intercellular lipids (sphingolipids) in cornified envelope cells and to find the relationships between them.

Transepidermal water loss (TEWL) is an indicator used to evaluate the barrier functions of the cornified envelope via noninvasive measurement. Although the barrier functions can also be evaluated using the transdermal absorptivity of substances, this is not universally used due to the limitations of the detection method.

The cornified envelope is the final product of epidermal turnover,[*] and the outermost cornified envelope that comes off as dead skin cells can easily be obtained without hurting the experimental subjects. For instance, whether the epidermal turnover is smooth or not can be checked using an adhesive transparent tape, and the rate of epidermal turnover can be determined from the magnitude of the dispersed cornified envelope cells. Furthermore, the physiologically active substances or enzyme activity in cornified envelope samples can be also measured. For instance, by measuring interleukin (a peptide responsible for the signal transduction between immunocompetent cells that direct cell proliferation and differentiation and protein synthesis) and related cytokines (biologically active factors that are involved in intercellular interactions such as the expression and regulation of immune responses), mild inflammation on the skin can be evaluated.

### 26.4.4  The role of cornified envelope cells as a barrier

The architecture of the cornified envelope demonstrates a block-and-mortar analogy in which flat envelope cells correspond to blocks and intercellular lipids correspond to mortar (Figure 26.15).

The cornified envelope cells are filled with keratin fibers and contain NMF, which are mainly composed of amino acids.

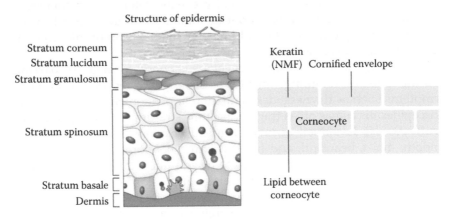

**Figure 26.15** Structure of the stratum corneum.

---

[*] *Turnover:* A phenomenon for various living body constituents to be replaced in the dynamic steady state with no change in the total quantity as the decomposition and synthesis progress at the same constant rate.

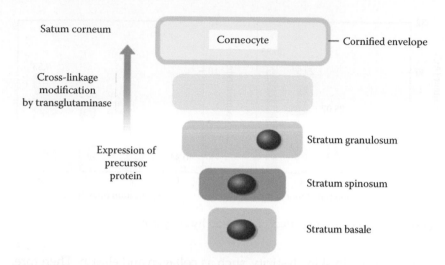

*Figure 26.16* Corneocyte formation process.

Meanwhile, intercellular lipids are in lamellar (thin film) structures formed by crystals composed of ceramide (a common structural unit of natural sphingolipids), cholesterol, and free fatty acids. The barrier functions can greatly vary with quantitative or qualitative changes in these intercellular lipids or with the loss of the polarity (Figure 26.16).

### 26.4.5 Functional cosmetics for the improvement of skin barriers made from the enzymatic hydrolysate products of cod skin

Recently, due to the depletion of land-derived resources, attempts have been made to explore the use of substances derived from living marine organisms to develop skin beauty care products. Collagen is the most important protein that constitutes the skin and plays a key role in maintaining the elasticity of the skin. Therefore, collagen per se has long been used as a cosmetic material for maintaining skin elasticity and moisture.

Cod skin was enzymatically hydrolyzed into low molecular hydrolysates that can be absorbed in the body and developed into functional materials that can be used for improving the skin's barrier properties and moisturize.

The enzymatic degradation products obtained from cod skin showed reactive oxygen and free radical scavenging activity and suppressed water loss in a dose-dependent manner. Besides, they increased the expression of the hyaluronan synthase gene, which is responsible for the synthesis of hyaluronic acid, which is an essential factor for maintaining skin moisture and elasticity. In addition, they also increased the expression of

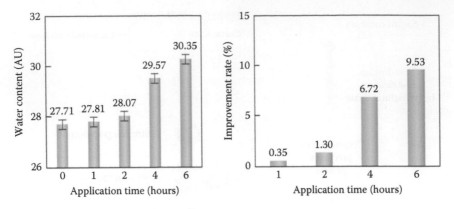

***Figure 26.17*** Moisturizing effect of cod skin hydrolysate.

factors involved in skin elasticity, such as collagen and elastin. Therefore, the enzymatic degradation products are said to be helpful in retaining the skin elasticity.

The application of enzymatically degraded cod skin elicited an up to 30% increase in the moisture content of the skin in females (Figure 26.17).

Specifically, in most of the female subjects, it prevented trans-epidermal water loss in the second week of use, indicating the efficacy of the sample in protecting and improving the skin barrier. The skin moisture content remarkably increased in two weeks of the application of the sample as compared with before application.

In addition, the skin elasticity gradually increased after one week of use (Figure 26.18). The enzymatic hydrolysate derived from cod skin is a byproduct of the fish processing industry. Therefore, the production

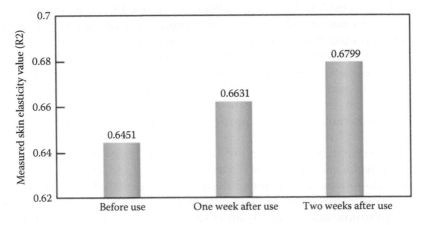

***Figure 26.18*** Skin elasticity-improving effects of cod skin hydrolysate.

process is very simple and cost-effective. In addition, the enzyme hydroly-sate increased the expression of those factors that play the most important roles in moisturizing and maintaining skin elasticity, and relevant clinical trials also showed the presence of an increased elasticity and moisture content of the skin. Therefore, the enzyme hydrolysate obtained from cod skin has a tremendous potential to help in retaining the skin's moisture and can be used as a high added-value cosmetic functional ingredient.

# References

Abe, S., Ishihara, K., Adachi, M. et al. (2006). Professional oral care reduces influenza infection in elderly. *Archives of Gerontology and Geriatrics*, 43, 157–164.

Ahn, B.-N., Kim, J.-A., Himaya, S., Bak, S.-S., Kong, C.-S., and Kim, S.-K. (2012). Chitooligosaccharides attenuate UVB-induced damages in human dermal fibroblasts. *Naunyn-Schmiedeberg's Archives of Pharmacology*, 385, 95–102.

Ahn, B.-N., Kim, J.-A., Kong, C.-S., Seo, Y., and Kim, S.-K. (2012). Protective effect of (2′ S)-columbianetin from *Corydalis heterocarpa* on UVB-induced keratinocyte damage. *Journal of Photochemistry and Photobiology B: Biology*, 109, 20–27.

Ahn, B. N., Kim, J., Kong, C. S., Seo, Y., and Kim, S.-K. (2013). Photoprotective effect of libanoridin isolated from *Corydalis heterocarpa* on UVB stressed human keratinocyte cells. *Experimental Dermatology*, 22, 155–157.

Alderman, M. H., Madhavan, S., Cohen, H., Sealey, J. E., and Laragh, J. H. (1995). Low urinary sodium is associated with greater risk of myocardial infarction among treated hypertensive men. *Hypertension*, 25, 1144–1152.

Anand, B. K. and Brobeck, J. R. (1951). Hypothalamic control of food intake in rats and cats. *The Yale Journal of Biology and Medicine*, 24, 123.

Artan, M., Li, Y., Karadeniz, F., Lee, S.-H., Kim, M.-M., and Kim, S.-K. (2008). Anti-HIV-1 activity of phloroglucinol derivative, 6, 6′-bieckol, from *Ecklonia cava*. *Bioorganic and Medicinal Chemistry*, 16, 7921–7926.

Athukorala, Y., Lee, K.-W., Kim, S.-K., and Jeon, Y.-J. (2007). Anticoagulant activity of marine green and brown algae collected from Jeju Island in Korea. *Bioresource Technology*, 98, 1711–1716.

Atsuko, T., Toshio, O., Makoto, T., and Tadashi, K. (1991). Possible origin of extremely high contents of vitamin $D_3$ in some kinds of fish liver. *Comparative Biochemistry and Physiology Part A: Physiology*, 100, 483–487.

Azuma, K., Ifuku, S., Osaki, T., Saimoto, H., and Okamoto, Y. (2016). Chitin derivatives as functional foods. In Kim, S.-K. (Ed.), *Marine Glycobiology*, pp. 459–468, CRC Press, Boca Raton, FL.

Bak, S.-S., Sung, Y. K., and Kim, S.-K. (2014). 7–Phloroeckol promotes hair growth on human follicles *in vitro*. *Naunyn-Schmiedeberg's Archives of Pharmacology*, 387, 789–793.

Bak, S., Ahn, B., Kim, J., Shin, S., Kim, J., Kim, M., Sung, Y., and Kim, S. (2013). *Ecklonia cava* promotes hair growth. *Clinical and Experimental Dermatology*, 38, 904–910.

Bang, J. K., Lee, J. H., Murugan, R. N., Lee, S. G., Do, H., Koh, H. Y., Shim, H.-E., Kim, H.-C., and Kim, H. J. (2013). Antifreeze peptides and glycopeptides, and their derivatives: Potential uses in biotechnology. *Marine Drugs*, 11, 2013–2041.

Bhatnagar, I. and Kim, S.-K. (2010). Marine antitumor drugs: Status, shortfalls and strategies. *Marine Drugs*, 8, 2702–2720.

Bjorksten, B., Naaber, P., Sepp, E., and Mikelsaar, M. (1999). The intestinal microflora in allergic Estonian and Swedish 2-year-old children. *Clinical and Experimental Allergy*, 29, 342–346.

Budtz-Jörgensen, E. and Bertram, U. (1970). Denture stomatitis I. The etiology in relation to trauma and infection. *Acta Odontologica Scandinavica*, 28, 71–92.

Byun, H.-G. and Kim, S.-K. (2001). Purification and characterization of angiotensin I converting enzyme (ACE) inhibitory peptides from Alaska pollack (*Theragra chalcogramma*) skin. *Process Biochemistry*, 36, 1155–1162.

Byun, H.-G. and Kim, S.-K. (2002). Structure and activity of angiotensin I converting enzyme inhibitory peptides derived from Alaskan pollack skin. *BMB Reports*, 35, 239–243.

Byun, H.-G., Kim, Y.-T., Park, P.-J., Lin, X., and Kim, S.-K. (2005). Chitooligosaccharides as a novel β-secretase inhibitor. *Carbohydrate Polymers*, 61, 198–202.

Cantin, A. M. (1994). Taurine modulation of hypochlorous acid-induced lung epithelial cell injury *in vitro*. Role of anion transport. *Journal of Clinical Investigation*, 93, 606–614.

Careaga, V. P. and Maier, M. S. (2015). Cytotoxic triterpene glycosides from sea cucumbers. In Kim, S.-K. (Ed.), *Handbook of Anticancer Drugs from Marine Origin*, pp. 515–528, Springer International Publishing, Cham, Switzerland.

Cha, S. H., Ko, S. C., Kim, D., and Jeon, Y. J. (2011). Screening of marine algae for potential tyrosinase inhibitor: Those inhibitors reduced tyrosinase activity and melanin synthesis in zebrafish. *The Journal of Dermatology*, 38, 354–363.

Chang, K. H. and Kim, J. M. (2001). Characteristics of HIV infection/AIDS in Korea. *The Korean Journal of Internal Medicine*, 16, 1.

Chen, T. T., Lin, C.-M., Chen, M. J., Lo, J. H., Chiou, P. P., Gong, H.-Y., Wu, J.-L., Chen, M. H.-C., and Yarish, C. (2015). Transgenic technology in marine organisms. In Kim, S.-K. (Ed.), *Springer Handbook of Marine Biotechnology*, pp. 387–412, Springer-Verlag, Berlin, Germany.

Cho, S. Y. (2014). Diagonosis and remedy of athlet's foot. *Drug Information*, 468, 13–18.

Cho, Y.-S., Jung, W.-K., Kim, J.-A., Choi, I.-W., and Kim, S.-K. (2009). Beneficial effects of fucoidan on osteoblastic MG-63 cell differentiation. *Food Chemistry*, 116, 990–994.

Crawford, M. and Marsh, D. (2002). Nutrition and evolution: A thumbs down book review. https://www.westonaprice.org/nutrition-and-evolution-by-michael-crawford-and-david-marsh/.

Cruz, C. F., Costa, C., Gomes, A. C., Matamá, T., and Cavaco-Paulo, A. (2016). Human hair and the impact of cosmetic procedures: A review on cleansing and shape-modulating cosmetics. *Cosmetics*, 3, 26.

Dahl, L. K. and Love, R. (1954). Evidence for relationship between sodium (chloride) intake and human essential hypertension. *AMA Archives of Internal Medicine*, 94, 525–531.

Demmer, R. T., Jacobs, D. R., and Desvarieux, M. (2008). Periodontal disease and incident type 2 diabetes. *Diabetes Care*, 31, 1373–1379.

Dewapriya, P. and Kim, S.-K. (2014). Marine microorganisms: An emerging avenue in modern nutraceuticals and functional foods. *Food Research International*, 56, 115–125.

Dobbs, R., Sawers, C., Thompson, F., Manyika, J., Woetzel, J., Child, P., McKenna, S., and Spatharou, A. (2014). How the world could better fight obesity. *McKinsey Global Institute*. https://www.mckinsey.com/industries/healthcare-systems-and-services/our-insights/how-the-world-could-better-fight-obesity.

Ekiken, K. (貝原益軒). (1977). Curing lesson (養生訓). pp. 57–58, Chuokoron-Shinsha.

Eom, S.-H., Kim, Y.-M., and Kim, S.-K. (2012). Antimicrobial effect of phlorotannins from marine brown algae. *Food and Chemical Toxicology*, 50, 3251–3255.

Eom, S. H., Lee, S. H., Yoon, N. Y., Jung, W. K., Jeon, Y. J., Kim, S. K., Lee, M. S., and Kim, Y. M. (2012). α-Glucosidase-and α-amylase-inhibitory activities of phlorotannins from *Eisenia bicyclis*. *Journal of the Science of Food and Agriculture*, 92, 2084–2090.

Eom, T.-K., Kong, C.-S., Byun, H.-G., Jung, W.-K., and Kim, S.-K. (2010). Lipase catalytic synthesis of diacylglycerol from tuna oil and its anti-obesity effect in C57BL/6J mice. *Process Biochemistry*, 45, 738–743.

Freeman, T. C., Ivens, A., Baillie, J. K. et al. (2012). A gene expression Atlas of the domestic pig. *BMC Biology*, 10(90070), 1–21.

Fusetani, N. (2010). Biotechnological potential of marine natural products. *Pure and Applied Chemistry*, 82, 17–26.

Gulliford, T., English, J., Colston, K., Menday, P., Moller, S., and Coombes, R. (1998). A phase I study of the vitamin D analogue EB 1089 in patients with advanced breast and colorectal cancer. *British Journal of Cancer*, 78, 6–10.

Hachimura, S. (2008). Mechanisms of suppression of allergy by lactic acid bacteria. *Bioindustry*, 25, 48–53.

Hayashi, Y., Yamauchi, M., Kim, S.-K., and Kusaoke, H. (2014). Biomaterials: Chitosan and collagen for regenerative medicine. *BioMed Research International*, 2014, 1.

Heo, S.-J., Ko, S.-C., Cha, S.-H., Kang, D.-H., Park, H.-S., Choi, Y.-U., Kim, D., Jung, W.-K., and Jeon, Y.-J. (2009). Effect of phlorotannins isolated from *Ecklonia cava* on melanogenesis and their protective effect against photo-oxidative stress induced by UV-B radiation. *Toxicology In Vitro*, 23, 1123–1130.

Heo, S.-J., Park, P.-J., Park, E.-J., Kim, S.-K., and Jeon, Y.-J. (2005). Antioxidant activity of enzymatic extracts from a brown seaweed *Ecklonia cava* by electron spin resonance spectrometry and comet assay. *European Food Research and Technology*, 221, 41–47.

Hideo, K. (2001). Hypertension and fisheries products. In Masakatsu, Y. (Ed.), *Health Functional Activities of Seafoods*, pp. 58–67, Kouseisha-Kouseika, Tokyo, Japan.

Hideo, K., Michiko, K., and Minoru, H. (2001). Osteoporosis and fisheries products. In Masakatsu, Y. (Ed.), *Health Functional Activities of Seafoods*, pp. 42–57, Kouseisha-Kouseikaku, Tokyo, Japan.

Himaya, S., Ngo, D.-H., Ryu, B., and Kim, S.-K. (2012). An active peptide purified from gastrointestinal enzyme hydrolysate of Pacific cod skin gelatin attenuates angiotensin-1 converting enzyme (ACE) activity and cellular oxidative stress. *Food Chemistry*, 132, 1872–1882.

Himaya, S., Ryu, B., Ngo, D.-H., and Kim, S.-K. (2012). Peptide isolated from Japanese flounder skin gelatin protects against cellular oxidative damage. *Journal of Agricultural and Food Chemistry*, 60, 9112–9119.

Himaya, S., Ryu, B., Qian, Z.-J., and Kim, S.-K. (2010). Sea cucumber, *Stichopus japonicus* ethyl acetate fraction modulates the lipopolysaccharide induced iNOS and COX-2 via MAPK signaling pathway in murine macrophages. *Environmental Toxicology and Pharmacology*, 30, 68–75.

Hirao, T. (2011). Evaluation of cornified envelope involved in barrier function of the stratum corneum. *Bioindustry*, 28, 7–14.

Hoang, V. L. and Kim, S.-K. (2013). Antimicrobial peptides from marine sources. *Current Protein and Peptide Science*, 14, 205–211.

Hong, H. C. (2015). Diagnosis and remedy of insomnia. *Drug Information Journal*, 477–482.

Huang, R., Mendis, E., Rajapakse, N., and Kim, S.-K. (2006). Strong electronic charge as an important factor for anticancer activity of chitooligosaccharides (COS). *Life Sciences*, 78, 2399–2408.

Huang, R., Rajapakse, N., and Kim, S.-K. (2006). Structural factors affecting radical scavenging activity of chitooligosaccharides (COS) and its derivatives. *Carbohydrate Polymers*, 63, 122–129.

Je, J.-Y., Cho, Y.-S., and Kim, S.-K. (2006). Cytotoxic activities of water-soluble chitosan derivatives with different degree of deacetylation. *Bioorganic and Medicinal Chemistry Letters*, 16, 2122–2126.

Je, J.-Y. and Kim, S.-K. (2005). Water-soluble chitosan derivatives as a BACE1 inhibitor. *Bioorganic and Medicinal Chemistry*, 13, 6551–6555.

Je, J.-Y. and Kim, S.-K. (2006a). Antimicrobial action of novel chitin derivative. *Biochimica et Biophysica Acta (BBA)-General Subjects*, 1760, 104–109.

Je, J.-Y. and Kim, S.-K. (2006b). Chitosan derivatives killed bacteria by disrupting the outer and inner membrane. *Journal of Agricultural and Food Chemistry*, 54, 6629–6633.

Je, J.-Y., Park, P.-J., and Kim, S.-K. (2004a). Free radical scavenging properties of hetero-chitooligosaccharides using an ESR spectroscopy. *Food and Chemical Toxicology*, 42, 381–387.

Je, J.-Y., Park, P.-J., and Kim, S.-K. (2004b). Radical scavenging activity of hetero-chitooligosaccharides. *European Food Research and Technology*, 219, 60–65.

Je, J.-Y., Park, P.-J., and Kim, S.-K. (2005). Antioxidant activity of a peptide isolated from Alaska pollack (*Theragra chalcogramma*) frame protein hydrolysate. *Food Research International*, 38, 45–50.

Je, J.-Y., Park, P.-J., Kwon, J. Y., and Kim, S.-K. (2004). A novel angiotensin I converting enzyme inhibitory peptide from Alaska pollack (*Theragra chalcogramma*) frame protein hydrolysate. *Journal of Agricultural and Food Chemistry*, 52, 7842–7845.

Je, J. Y., Park, P. J., Kim, B., and Kim, S. K. (2006). Antihypertensive activity of chitin derivatives. *Biopolymers*, 83, 250–254.

Jensen, I. J., Eilertsen, K. E., Mæhre, H. K., Elvevoll, E. O., and Larsen, R. (2013). Health effects of antioxidative and antihypertensive peptides from marine resources. In Kim, S.-K. (Ed.), *Marine Proteins and Peptides: Biological Activities and Applications*, pp. 297–322, Wiley-Blackwell, Hoboken, NJ.

Jeon, Y.-J., Byun, H.-G., and Kim, S.-K. (1999). Improvement of functional properties of cod frame protein hydrolysates using ultrafiltration membranes. *Process Biochemistry*, 35, 471–478.

Jeon, Y.-J. and Kim, S.-K. (2000a). Continuous production of chitooligosaccharides using a dual reactor system. *Process Biochemistry*, 35, 623–632.

Jeon, Y.-J. and Kim, S.-K. (2000b). Production of chitooligosaccharides using an ultrafiltration membrane reactor and their antibacterial activity. *Carbohydrate Polymers*, 41, 133–141.

Jeon, Y.-J. and Kim, S.-K. (2002). Antitumor activity of chitosan oligosaccharides produced in ultrafiltration membrane reactor system. *Journal of Microbiology and Biotechnology*, 12, 503–507.

Jeon, Y.-J., Park, P.-J., and Kim, S.-K. (2001). Antimicrobial effect of chitooligosaccharides produced by bioreactor. *Carbohydrate Polymers*, 44, 71–76.

Jeon, Y.-J., Shahidi, F., and Kim, S.-K. (2000). Preparation of chitin and chitosan oligomers and their applications in physiological functional foods. *Food Reviews International*, 16, 159–176.

Jing, K. and Lim, K. (2013). Potent anticancer actions of omega-3 polyunsaturated fatty acids of marine nutraceuticals. In Kim, S.-K. (Ed.), *Marine Nutraceuticals*, pp. 199–232, CRC Press, Boca Raton, FL.

Jo, H.-Y., Jung, W.-K., and Kim, S.-K. (2008). Purification and characterization of a novel anticoagulant peptide from marine echiuroid worm, *Urechis unicinctus*. *Process Biochemistry*, 43, 179–184.

Jung, W.-K., Ahn, Y.-W., Lee, S.-H., Choi, Y. H., Kim, S.-K., Yea, S. S., Choi, I., Park, S.-G., Seo, S.-K., and Lee, S.-W. (2009). *Ecklonia cava* ethanolic extracts inhibit lipopolysaccharide-induced cyclooxygenase-2 and inducible nitric oxide synthase expression in BV2 microglia via the MAP kinase and NF-κB pathways. *Food and Chemical Toxicology*, 47, 410–417.

Jung, W.-K., Athukorala, Y., Lee, Y.-J., Cha, S. H., Lee, C.-H., Vasanthan, T., Choi, K.-S., Yoo, S.-H., Kim, S.-K., and Jeon, Y.-J. (2007). Sulfated polysaccharide purified from *Ecklonia cava* accelerates antithrombin III-mediated plasma proteinase inhibition. *Journal of Applied Phycology*, 19, 425–430.

Jung, W.-K., Je, J.-Y., Kim, H.-J., and Kim, S.-K. (2002). A novel anticoagulant protein from *Scapharca broughtonii*. *BMB Reports*, 35, 199–205.

Jung, W.-K., Karawita, R., Heo, S.-J., Lee, B.-J., Kim, S.-K., and Jeon, Y.-J. (2006). Recovery of a novel Ca-binding peptide from Alaska Pollack (*Theragra chalcogramma*) backbone by pepsinolytic hydrolysis. *Process Biochemistry*, 41, 2097–2100.

Jung, W.-K. and Kim, S.-K. (2009). Isolation and characterisation of an anticoagulant oligopeptide from blue mussel, *Mytilus edulis*. *Food Chemistry*, 117, 687–692.

Jung, W.-K., Lee, B.-J., and Kim, S.-K. (2006). Fish-bone peptide increases calcium solubility and bioavailability in ovariectomised rats. *British Journal of Nutrition*, 95, 124–128.

Jung, W.-K., Lee, D.-Y., Choi, Y. H., Yea, S. S., Choi, I., Park, S.-G., Seo, S.-K., Lee, S.-W., Lee, C.-M., and Kim, S.-K. (2008a). Caffeic acid phenethyl ester attenuates allergic airway inflammation and hyperresponsiveness in murine model of ovalbumin-induced asthma. *Life Sciences*, 82, 797–805.

Jung, W.-K., Lee, D.-Y., Kim, J.-H., Choi, I., Park, S.-G., Seo, S.-K., Lee, S.-W., Lee, C.-M., Park, Y.-M., and Jeon, Y.-J. (2008b). Anti-inflammatory activity of caffeic acid phenethyl ester (CAPE) extracted from *Rhodiola sacra* against lipopolysaccharide-induced inflammatory responses in mice. *Process Biochemistry*, 43, 783–787.

Jung, W.-K., Moon, S.-H., and Kim, S.-K. (2006). Effect of chitooligosaccharides on calcium bioavailability and bone strength in ovariectomized rats. *Life Sciences*, 78, 970–976.

Kalimuthu, S. and Kim, S.-K. (2013). Cell survival and apoptosis signaling as therapeutic target for cancer: Marine bioactive compounds. *International Journal of Molecular Sciences*, 14, 2334–2354.

Kalliomäki, M., Salminen, S., Arvilommi, H., Kero, P., Koskinen, P., and Isolauri, E. (2001). Probiotics in primary prevention of atopic disease: A randomised placebo-controlled trial. *Lancet*, 357(9262), 1076–1079.

Kalliomäki, M., Salminen, S., Poussa, T., Arvilommi, H., and Isolauri, E. (2003). Probiotics and prevention of atopic disease: 4-year follow-up of a randomised placebo-controlled trial. *Lancet*, 361, 1869–1871.

Kamio, N., Imai, K., and Ochiai, K. (2015). Relationship between oral bacteria and Influenza virus. *Bioindustry*, 32, 25–29.

Kang, M.-C., Kang, N., Kim, S.-Y., Lima, I. S., Ko, S.-C., Kim, Y.-T., Kim, Y.-B., Jeung, H.-D., Choi, K.-S., and Jeon, Y.-J. (2016). Popular edible seaweed, *Gelidium amansii* prevents against diet-induced obesity. *Food and Chemical Toxicology*, 90, 181–187.

Karadeniz, F., Artan, M., Kong, C.-S., and Kim, S.-K. (2010). Chitooligosaccharides protect pancreatic β-cells from hydrogen peroxide-induced deterioration. *Carbohydrate Polymers*, 82, 143–147.

Karadeniz, F., Kang, K.-H., Park, J. W., Park, S.-J., and Kim, S.-K. (2014). Anti-HIV-1 activity of phlorotannin derivative 8, 4'-dieckol from Korean brown alga *Ecklonia cava*. *Bioscience, Biotechnology, and Biochemistry*, 78, 1151–1158.

Karadeniz, F., Mustafa, Z. K., Kong, C.-S., and Kim, S.-K. (2011). *In vitro* anti-HIV-1 activity of the aqueous extract of *Asterina pectinifera*. *Current HIV Research*, 9, 95–102.

Kato, H., Taguchi, T., Okuda, H., Kondo, M., and Takara, M. (1994). Antihypertensive effect of chitosan in rats and humans. *Journal of Traditional Medicine*, 11, 198–205.

Kato, H. et al. (2001). Osteoporosis and fisheries products. In Masakatsu, Y. (Ed.), *Health Functional Activities of Seafoods*, pp. 42–56, Kouseisha-Kouseikakaku, Tokyo, Japan.

Khor, E. (2010). Medical applications of chitin and chitosan. In Kim, S.-K. (Ed.), *Chitin, Chitosan, Oligosaccharides and Their Derivatives*, pp. 405–413, CRC Press, Boca Raton, FL.

Kibo, H. (1994). *Medical Applications of Chitin and Chitosan*, Gihoto Publishing, Tokyo, Japan.

Kifune, K. (1994). *Medical Applications of Chitin and Chitosan*, pp. 71–104, Ginodo Shuppan, Tokyo, Japan.

Kim, I., Yoo, M., Seo, J., Park, S., Na, H., Lee, H., Kim, S., and Cho, C. (2007). Evaluation of semi-interpenetrating polymer networks composed of chitosan and poloxamer for wound dressing application. *International Journal of Pharmaceutics*, 341, 35–43.

Kim, J.-A., Ahn, B.-N., Kong, C.-S., and Kim, S.-K. (2011). Anti-inflammatory action of sulfated glucosamine on cytokine regulation in LPS-activated PMA-differentiated THP-1 macrophages. *Inflammation Research*, 60, 1131–1138.

Kim, J.-A., Ahn, B.-N., Kong, C.-S., and Kim, S.-K. (2012). Chitooligomers inhibit UV-A-induced photoaging of skin by regulating TGF-β/Smad signaling cascade. *Carbohydrate Polymers*, 88, 490–495.

Kim, J. A., Ahn, B. N., Kong, C. S., and Kim, S. K. (2013). The chromene sargachromanol E inhibits ultraviolet A-induced ageing of skin in human dermal fibroblasts. *British Journal of Dermatology*, 168, 968–976.

Kim, J.-A. and Kim, S.-K. (2013). Bioactive peptides from marine sources as potential anti-inflammatory therapeutics. *Current Protein and Peptide Science*, 14, 177–182.

Kim, J.-A., Kong, C.-S., and Kim, S.-K. (2010). Effect of *Sargassum thunbergii* on ROS mediated oxidative damage and identification of polyunsaturated fatty acid components. *Food and Chemical Toxicology*, 48, 1243–1249.

Kim, J.-A., Kong, C.-S., Pyun, S. Y., and Kim, S.-K. (2010). Phosphorylated glucosamine inhibits the inflammatory response in LPS-stimulated PMA-differentiated THP-1 cells. *Carbohydrate Research*, 345, 1851–1855.

Kim, J.-A., Kong, C.-S., Seo, Y.-W., and Kim, S.-K. (2010). *Sargassum thunbergii* extract inhibits MMP-2 and-9 expressions related with ROS scavenging in HT1080 cells. *Food Chemistry*, 120, 418–425.

Kim, K.-N., Ahn, G., Heo, S.-J., Kang, S.-M., Kang, M.-C., Yang, H.-M., Kim, D., Roh, S. W., Kim, S.-K., and Jeon, B.-T. (2013). Inhibition of tumor growth *in vitro* and *in vivo* by fucoxanthin against melanoma B16F10 cells. *Environmental Toxicology and Pharmacology*, 35, 39–46.

Kim, M.-M. and Kim, S.-K. (2006). Chitooligosaccharides inhibit activation and expression of matrix metalloproteinase-2 in human dermal fibroblasts. *FEBS Letters*, 580, 2661–2666.

Kim, M.-M. and Kim, S.-K. (2010). Effect of phloroglucinol on oxidative stress and inflammation. *Food and Chemical Toxicology*, 48, 2925–2933.

Kim, M.-M., Van Ta, Q., Mendis, E., Rajapakse, N., Jung, W.-K., Byun, H.-G., Jeon, Y.-J., and Kim, S.-K. (2006). Phlorotannins in *Ecklonia cava* extract inhibit matrix metalloproteinase activity. *Life Sciences*, 79, 1436–1443.

Kim, M. M., Mendis, E., Rajapakse, N., and Kim, S.-K. (2007). Glucosamine sulfate promotes osteoblastic differentiation of MG-63 cells via anti-inflammatory effect. *Bioorganic and Medicinal Chemistry Letters*, 17, 1938–1942.

Kim, M. M., Mendis, E., Rajapakse, N., Lee, S. H., and Kim, S. K. (2009). Effect of spongin derived from *Hymeniacidon sinapium* on bone mineralization. *Journal of Biomedical Materials Research Part B: Applied Biomaterials*, 90, 540–546.

Kim, M. M., Rajapakse, N., and Kim, S. K. (2009). Anti-inflammatory effect of *Ishige okamurae* ethanolic extract via inhibition of NF-κB transcription factor in RAW 264.7 cells. *Phytotherapy Research*, 23, 628–634.

Kim, S.-K. (2001a). Effect of antimicrobial activity by chitosan oligosaccharide N-conjugated with asparagine. *Journal of Microbiology and Biotechnology*, 11, 281–286.

Kim, S. K. (2001b). *Chitosan Oligosaccharides Can Revive You*, pp. 64–75, Taeyl Publisher, Seoul, South Korea.

Kim, S.-K. and Bak, S.-S. (2011). Hair biology and care product ingredients from marine organisms. In Kim, S.-K. (Ed.), *Marine Cosmeceuticals*, pp. 201–210, CRC Press, Boca Raton, FL.

Kim, S.-K., Kim, Y.-T., Byun, H.-G., Nam, K.-S., Joo, D.-S., and Shahidi, F. (2001). Isolation and characterization of antioxidative peptides from gelatin hydrolysate of Alaska pollack skin. *Journal of Agricultural and Food Chemistry*, 49, 1984–1989.

Kim, S.-K. and Kong, C.-S. (2010). Anti-adipogenic effect of dioxinodehydroeckol via AMPK activation in 3T3-L1 adipocytes. *Chemico-Biological Interactions*, 186, 24–29.

Kim, S.-K., Lee, D.-Y., Jung, W.-K., Kim, J.-H., Choi, I., Park, S.-G., Seo, S.-K., Lee, S.-W., Lee, C. M., and Yea, S. S. (2008). Effects of *Ecklonia cava* ethanolic extracts on airway hyperresponsiveness and inflammation in a murine asthma model: Role of suppressor of cytokine signaling. *Biomedicine and Pharmacotherapy*, 62, 289–296.

Kim, S.-K. and Mendis, E. (2006). Bioactive compounds from marine processing byproducts–A review. *Food Research International*, 39, 383–393.

Kim, S.-K., Park, P.-J., Jung, W.-K., Byun, H.-G., Mendis, E., and Cho, Y.-I. (2005). Inhibitory activity of phosphorylated chitooligosaccharides on the formation of calcium phosphate. *Carbohydrate Polymers*, 60, 483–487.

Kim, S.-K. and Rajapakse, N. (2005). Enzymatic production and biological activities of chitosan oligosaccharides (COS): A review. *Carbohydrate Polymers*, 62, 357–368.

Kim, S.-K., Ravichandran, Y. D., and Kong, C.-S. (2012). Applications of calcium and its supplement derived from marine organisms. *Critical Reviews in Food Science and Nutrition*, 52, 469–474.

Kim, S.-K., Vo, T.-S., and Ngo, D.-H. (2012). The immunomodulatory effect of marine algae on allergic response. In Kim, S.-K. (Ed.), *Marine Pharmacognosy*, pp. 101–106, CRC Press, Boca Raton, FL.

Kim, S.-K. and Wijesekara, I. (2010). Development and biological activities of marine-derived bioactive peptides: A review. *Journal of Functional Foods*, 2, 1–9.

Kim, S. K. (2013). The possible roles of chitosan and its derivatives in cardiovascular health; an overview. *Journal of Chitin and Chitosan*, 18, 137–143.

Kim, S. K., Vo, T. S., and Ngo, D. H. (2013). Marine algae: Pharmacological values and anti-inflammatory effects. In Kim, S.-K. (Ed.), *Marine Pharmacognosy*, pp. 273–280, CRC Press, Boca Raton, FL.

Kim, T.-Y., Jin, C.-Y., Kim, G.-Y., Choi, I.-W., Jeong, Y. K., Nam, T.-J., Kim, S.-K., and Choi, Y. H. (2009). Ethyl alcohol extracts of *Hizikia fusiforme* sensitize AGS human gastric adenocarcinoma cells to tumor necrosis factor-related apoptosis-inducing ligand-mediated apoptosis. *Journal of Medicinal Food*, 12, 782–787.

Kim, Y. J., Han, J. W., So, Y. S., Seo, J. Y., Kim, K. Y., and Kim, K. W. (2014). Prevalence and trends of dementia in Korea: A systematic review and meta-analysis. *Journal of Korean Medical Science*, 29, 903–912.

Ko, S.-C., Lee, S.-H., Ahn, G., Kim, K.-N., Cha, S.-H., Kim, S.-K., Jeon, B.-T., Park, P.-J., Lee, K.-W., and Jeon, Y.-J. (2012). Effect of enzyme-assisted extract of *Sargassum coreanum* on induction of apoptosis in HL-60 tumor cells. *Journal of Applied Phycology*, 24, 675–684.

Kondo, N. (2008). The reasons for increasing the numbers of allergic patients. *Bioindustry*, 25, 7–14.

Kong, C.-S., Kim, J.-A., Ahn, B.-N., and Kim, S.-K. (2011). Potential effect of phloroglucinol derivatives from *Ecklonia cava* on matrix metalloproteinase expression and the inflammatory profile in lipopolysaccharide-stimulated human THP-1 macrophages. *Fisheries Science*, 77, 867–873.

Kong, C.-S., Kim, J.-A., Ahn, B.-N., Vo, T. S., Yoon, N.-Y., and Kim, S.-K. (2010). 1-(3′, 5′-dihydroxyphenoxy)-7-(2 ″, 4 ″, 6-trihydroxyphenoxy)-2, 4, 9-trihydroxydibenzo-1, 4-dioxin Inhibits adipocyte differentiation of 3T3-L1 fibroblasts. *Marine Biotechnology*, 12, 299–307.

Kong, C.-S., Kim, J.-A., Eom, T. K., and Kim, S.-K. (2010). Phosphorylated glucosamine inhibits adipogenesis in 3T3-L1 adipocytes. *The Journal of Nutritional Biochemistry*, 21, 438–443.

Kong, C.-S., Kim, J.-A., and Kim, S.-K. (2009). Anti-obesity effect of sulfated glucosamine by AMPK signal pathway in 3T3-L1 adipocytes. *Food and Chemical Toxicology*, 47, 2401–2406.

Kong, C.-S., Kim, J.-A., Yoon, N.-Y., and Kim, S.-K. (2009). Induction of apoptosis by phloroglucinol derivative from *Ecklonia cava* in MCF-7 human breast cancer cells. *Food and Chemical Toxicology*, 47, 1653–1658.

Kong, C.-S., Kim, Y. A., Kim, M.-M., Park, J.-S., Kim, J.-A., Kim, S.-K., Lee, B.-J., Nam, T. J., and Seo, Y. (2008). Flavonoid glycosides isolated from *Salicornia herbacea* inhibit matrix metalloproteinase in HT1080 cells. *Toxicology In Vitro*, 22, 1742–1748.

Korean Dermatological Association. (2014). *Textbook of Dermatology*, 6th ed., pp. 472–476, Daehaneuihak, Seoul.

Kurtz, T. W., Al-Bander, H. A., and Morris Jr, R. C. (1987). Salt-sensitive essential hypertension in men. *New England Journal of Medicine*, 317, 1043–1048.

Le, Q.-T., Li, Y., Qian, Z.-J., Kim, M.-M., and Kim, S.-K. (2009). Inhibitory effects of polyphenols isolated from marine alga *Ecklonia cava* on histamine release. *Process Biochemistry*, 44, 168–176.

Lee, K. S. and Suh, H.-S. (2012). Alzheimer's disease: Clinical trials and future perspectives. *Korean Journal of Psychopharmacology*, 23, 131–135.

Lee, S.-H., Choi, J.-I., Heo, S.-J., Park, M.-H., Park, P.-J., Jeon, B.-T., Kim, S.-K., Han, J.-S., and Jeon, Y.-J. (2012a). Diphlorethohydroxycarmalol isolated from Pae (*Ishige okamurae*) protects high glucose-induced damage in RINm5F pancreatic β cells via its antioxidant effects. *Food Science and Biotechnology*, 21, 239–246.

Lee, S.-H., Karadeniz, F., Kim, M.-M., and Kim, S.-K. (2008). Alpha-glucosidase and alpha-amylase inhibitory activities of phlorotannin derivatives from *Ecklonia cava*. *Journal of Biotechnology*, 136, S588.

Lee, S.-H., Min, K.-H., Han, J.-S., Lee, D.-H., Park, D.-B., Jung, W.-K., Park, P.-J., Jeon, B.-T., Kim, S.-K., and Jeon, Y.-J. (2012b). Effects of brown alga, *Ecklonia cava* on glucose and lipid metabolism in C57BL/KsJ-db/db mice, a model of type 2 diabetes mellitus. *Food and Chemical Toxicology*, 50, 575–582.

Lee, S.-H., Park, J.-S., Kim, S.-K., Ahn, C.-B., and Je, J.-Y. (2009). Chitooligosaccharides suppress the level of protein expression and acetylcholinesterase activity induced by Aβ 25–35 in PC12 cells. *Bioorganic and Medicinal Chemistry Letters*, 19, 860–862.

Lee, S.-H., Park, M.-H., Kang, S.-M., Ko, S.-C., Kang, M.-C., Cho, S., Park, P.-J., Jeon, B.-T., Kim, S.-K., and Han, J.-S. (2012c). Dieckol isolated from *Ecklonia cava* protects against high-glucose induced damage to rat insulinoma cells by reducing oxidative stress and apoptosis. *Bioscience, Biotechnology, and Biochemistry*, 76, 1445–1451.

Lee, S.-H., Qian, Z.-J., and Kim, S.-K. (2010). A novel angiotensin I converting enzyme inhibitory peptide from tuna frame protein hydrolysate and its antihypertensive effect in spontaneously hypertensive rats. *Food Chemistry*, 118, 96–102.

Lee, S.-H., Senevirathne, M., Ahn, C.-B., Kim, S.-K., and Je, J.-Y. (2009). Factors affecting anti-inflammatory effect of chitooligosaccharides in lipopolysaccharides-induced RAW264. 7 macrophage cells. *Bioorganic and Medicinal Chemistry Letters*, 19, 6655–6658.

Lee, S. G., Lee, J. H., Kang, S. H., and Kim, H. J. (2013). Marine antifreeze proteins: Types, functions and applications. In Kim, S.-K. (Ed.), *Marine Proteins and Peptides: Biological Activities and Applications*, pp. 667–694, Wiley-Blackwell, Hoboken, NJ.

Lee, S. H., Karadeniz, F., Kim, M. M., and Kim, S. K. (2009). α-Glucosidase and α-amylase inhibitory activities of phloroglucinal derivatives from edible marine brown alga, *Ecklonia cava*. *Journal of the Science of Food and Agriculture*, 89, 1552–1558.

Lee, W.-W., Ahn, G., Arachchillage, J. P. W., Kim, Y. M., Kim, S.-K., Lee, B.-J., and Jeon, Y.-J. (2011). A polysaccharide isolated from *Ecklonia cava* fermented by *Lactobacillus brevis* inhibits the inflammatory response by suppressing the activation of nuclear factor-κB in lipopolysaccharide-induced RAW 264.7 macrophages. *Journal of Medicinal Food*, 14, 1546–1553.

Li, S. (1590). *Ben cao gang mu (Compendium of Materia Medica)*. People's Health Publishing House, Beijing.

Li, Y.-X., Himaya, S., and Kim, S.-K. (2013). Triterpenoids of marine origin as anticancer agents. *Molecules*, 18, 7886–7909.

Li, Y.-X. and Kim, S.-K. (2011). Utilization of seaweed derived ingredients as potential antioxidants and functional ingredients in the food industry: An overview. *Food Science and Biotechnology*, 20, 1461–1466.

Li, Y.-X., Li, Y., Je, J.-Y., and Kim, S.-K. (2015). Dieckol as a novel anti-proliferative and anti-angiogenic agent and computational anti-angiogenic activity evaluation. *Environmental Toxicology and Pharmacology*, 39, 259–270.

Li, Y.-X., Li, Y., Lee, S.-H., Qian, Z.-J., and Kim, S.-K. (2009). Inhibitors of oxidation and matrix metalloproteinases, floridoside, and D-isofloridoside from marine red alga *Laurencia undulata*. *Journal of Agricultural and Food Chemistry*, 58, 578–586.

Li, Y.-X., Wijesekara, I., Li, Y., and Kim, S.-K. (2011). Phlorotannins as bioactive agents from brown algae. *Process Biochemistry*, 46, 2219–2224.

Li, Y., Lee, S.-H., Le, Q.-T., Kim, M.-M., and Kim, S.-K. (2008). Anti-allergic effects of phlorotannins on histamine release via binding inhibition between IgE and FcεRI. *Journal of Agricultural and Food Chemistry*, 56, 12073–12080.

Li, Y., Qian, Z.-J., Kim, M.-M., and Kim, S.-K. (2011). Cytotoxic activities of phlorethol and fucophlorethol derivatives isolated from *Laminariaceae Ecklonia cava*. *Journal of Food Biochemistry*, 35, 357–369.

Li, Y., Qian, Z.-J., Ryu, B., Lee, S.-H., Kim, M.-M., and Kim, S.-K. (2009). Chemical components and its antioxidant properties *in vitro*: An edible marine brown alga, *Ecklonia cava*. *Bioorganic and Medicinal Chemistry*, 17, 1963–1973.

Lim, J. Y., and Jegal, M. (2014). The recent research trend of hair loss prevent. *Korean Journal of Aesthetics and Cosmetology*, 12, 773–789.

Medical Observer. (2015). Increasing of domestic dimentia patients. *Korean Journal of Social Welfare Studies*. http://www.mohw.go.kr/react/al/sal0301vw.jsp?PAR_MENU_ID=04&MENU_ID=0403&CONT_SEQ=286138.

Melanie, A., Banks, D. W., Porter, W. G., and Martin, V. C. (1990). Effects of in vitro ozone exposure on peroxidative damage, membrane leakage, and taurine content of rat alveolar macrophages. *Toxicology and Applied Pharmacology*, 105(1), 55–65.

Mendis, E., Kim, M.-M., Rajapakse, N., and Kim, S.-K. (2007). An *in vitro* cellular analysis of the radical scavenging efficacy of chitooligosaccharides. *Life Sciences*, 80, 2118–2127.

Mendis, E., Kim, M.-M., Rajapakse, N., and Kim, S.-K. (2008). Suppression of cytokine production in lipopolysaccharide-stimulated mouse macrophages by novel cationic glucosamine derivative involves down-regulation of NF-κB and MAPK expressions. *Bioorganic and Medicinal Chemistry*, 16, 8390–8396.

Mendis, E., Kim, M.-M., Rajapakse, N., and Kim, S.-K. (2009). The inhibitory mechanism of a novel cationic glucosamine derivative against MMP-2 and MMP-9 expressions. *Bioorganic and Medicinal Chemistry Letters*, 19, 2755–2759.

Mendis, E., Rajapakse, N., and Kim, S.-K. (2005). Antioxidant properties of a radical-scavenging peptide purified from enzymatically prepared fish skin gelatin hydrolysate. *Journal of Agricultural and Food Chemistry*, 53, 581–587.

Ministry of Health and Welfare. (2014). Press release. Revised Act of long-term care insurance reflecting on introduction of special classification of dementia. http://www.mohw.go.kr/react/al/sal0301vw.jsp?PAR_MENU_ID=04&MENU_ID=0403&CONT_SEQ=286138.

Miyazaki, Y., Kikuchi, K., and Kusama, K. (2015). Oral microorganisms and cancer. *Bioindustry*, 32, 38–45.

Nam, Y. K., Noh, J. K., Cho, Y. S., Cho, H. J., Cho, K.-N., Kim, C. G., and Kim, D. S. (2001). Dramatically accelerated growth and extraordinary gigantism of transgenic mud loach *Misgurnus mizolepis*. *Transgenic Research*, 10, 353–362.

Nelson, R. G., Shlossman, M., Budding, L. M., Pettitt, D. J., Saad, M. F., Genco, R. J., and Knowler, W. C. (1990). Periodontal disease and NIDDM in Pima Indians. *Diabetes Care*, 13(8), 836–840.

Ngo, D.-H., Kang, K.-H., Jung, W.-K., Byun, H.-G., and Kim, S.-K. (2014). Protective effects of peptides from skate (*Okamejei kenojei*) skin gelatin against endothelial dysfunction. *Journal of Functional Foods*, 10, 243–251.

Ngo, D.-H., Kang, K.-H., Ryu, B., Vo, T.-S., Jung, W.-K., Byun, H.-G., and Kim, S.-K. (2015a). Angiotensin-I converting enzyme inhibitory peptides from antihypertensive skate (*Okamejei kenojei*) skin gelatin hydrolysate in spontaneously hypertensive rats. *Food Chemistry*, 174, 37–43.

Ngo, D.-H. and Kim, S.-K. (2013). Marine bioactive peptides as potential antioxidants. *Current Protein and Peptide Science*, 14, 189–198.

Ngo, D.-H., Ryu, B., and Kim, S.-K. (2014). Active peptides from skate (*Okamejei kenojei*) skin gelatin diminish angiotensin-I converting enzyme activity and intracellular free radical-mediated oxidation. *Food Chemistry*, 143, 246–255.

Ngo, D.-H., Ryu, B., Vo, T.-S., Himaya, S., Wijesekara, I., and Kim, S.-K. (2011). Free radical scavenging and angiotensin-I converting enzyme inhibitory peptides from Pacific cod (*Gadus macrocephalus*) skin gelatin. *International Journal of Biological Macromolecules*, 49, 1110–1116.

Ngo, D.-H., Vo, T.-S., Ngo, D.-N., Kang, K.-H., Je, J.-Y., Pham, H. N.-D., Byun, H.-G., and Kim, S.-K. (2015b). Biological effects of chitosan and its derivatives. *Food Hydrocolloids*, 51, 200–216.

Ngo, D.-H., Vo, T.-S., Ngo, D.-N., Wijesekara, I., and Kim, S.-K. (2012). Biological activities and potential health benefits of bioactive peptides derived from marine organisms. *International Journal of Biological Macromolecules*, 51, 378–383.

Ngo, D.-H., Wijesekara, I., Vo, T.-S., Van Ta, Q., and Kim, S.-K. (2011). Marine food-derived functional ingredients as potential antioxidants in the food industry: An overview. *Food Research International*, 44, 523–529.

Ngo, D.-N., Kim, M.-M., and Kim, S.-K. (2008). Chitin oligosaccharides inhibit oxidative stress in live cells. *Carbohydrate Polymers*, 74, 228–234.

Ngo, D.-N., Kim, M.-M., Qian, Z. J., Jung, W.-K., Lee, S. H., and Kim, S.-K. (2010). Free radical-scavenging activities of low molecular weight oligosaccharides lead to antioxidant effect in live cells. *Journal of Food Biochemistry*, 34, 161–177.

Ngo, D.-N., Lee, S.-H., Kim, M.-M., and Kim, S.-K. (2009). Production of chitin oligosaccharides with different molecular weights and their antioxidant effect in RAW 264.7 cells. *Journal of Functional Foods*, 1, 188–198.

Obinata, K., Maruyama, T., Hayashi, M., Watanabe, T., and Nittono, H. (1996). Effect of taurine on the fatty liver of children with simple obesity. In Huxtable, R. J., Azuma, J., Kuriyama, K., Nakagawa, M., and Baba, A. (Eds.), *Taurine 2. Advances in Experimental Medicine and Biology*, pp. 607–613, Springer, New York.

OECD Social Indicators. (2015). Society at a glance. https://data.oecd.org/society.htm.

Ohara, N., Hayashi, Y., Yamada, S., Kim, S.-K., Matsunaga, T., Yanagiguchi, K., and Ikeda, T. (2004). Early gene expression analyzed by cDNA microarray and RT-PCR in osteoblasts cultured with water-soluble and low molecular chitooligosaccharide. *Biomaterials*, 25, 1749–1754.

Ohayon, M. M. (2002). Epidemiology of insomnia: What we know and what we still need to learn. *Sleep Medicine Reviews*, 6, 97–111.

Ohayon, M. M. and Hong, S.-C. (2002). Prevalence of insomnia and associated factors in South Korea. *Journal of Psychosomatic Research*, 53, 593–600.

Okuda, H. (1994). Chitin and chitosan: Fundamental and pharmacology. *Pharmacy Newspaper Co*, pp. 18–35.

Okuda, H. (2001). Obesity and fisheries products. In Masakatsu, Y. (Ed.), *Health Functional Activities of Seafoods*, pp. 1–6, Kouseisha-Kouseikakaku, Tokyo, Japan.

Organization for Economic Co-Operation and Development. (2012). Obesity update 2012. http://www.oecd.org/health/49716427.pdf.

Pallela, R., Na-Young, Y., and Kim, S.-K. (2010). Anti-photoaging and photoprotective compounds derived from marine organisms. *Marine Drugs*, 8, 1189–1202.

Pangestuti, R., Bak, S.-S., and Kim, S.-K. (2011). Attenuation of pro-inflammatory mediators in LPS-stimulated BV2 microglia by chitooligosaccharides via the MAPK signaling pathway. *International Journal of Biological Macromolecules*, 49, 599–606.

Pangestuti, R. and Kim, S.-K. (2010). Neuroprotective properties of chitosan and its derivatives. *Marine Drugs*, 8, 2117–2128.

Pangestuti, R. and Kim, S.-K. (2011a). Biological activities and health benefit effects of natural pigments derived from marine algae. *Journal of Functional Foods*, 3, 255–266.

Pangestuti, R. and Kim, S.-K. (2011b). Neuroprotective effects of marine algae. *Marine Drugs*, 9, 803–818.

Pangestuti, R. and Kim, S.-K. (2013). Marine-derived bioactive materials for neuroprotection. *Food Science and Biotechnology*, 22, 1–12.

Pangestuti, R., Vo, T.-S., Ngo, D.-H., and Kim, S.-K. (2013). Fucoxanthin ameliorates inflammation and oxidative reponses in microglia. *Journal of Agricultural and Food Chemistry*, 61, 3876–3883.

Park, M. K., Park, K. Y., Li, K., Seo, S. J., and Hong, C. K. (2013). The short stature in atopic dermatitis patients: Are atopic children really small for their age? *Annals of Dermatology*, 25, 23–27.

Park, P.-J., Je, J.-Y., Byun, H.-G., Moon, S.-H., and Kim, S.-K. (2004). Antimicrobial activity of hetero-chitosans and their oligosaccharides with different molecular weights. *Journal of Microbiology and Biotechnology*, 14, 317–323.

Park, P.-J., Je, J.-Y., Jung, W.-K., Ahn, C.-B., and Kim, S.-K. (2004). Anticoagulant activity of heterochitosans and their oligosaccharide sulfates. *European Food Research and Technology*, 219, 529–533.

Park, P.-J., Je, J.-Y., and Kim, S.-K. (2003a). Angiotensin I converting enzyme (ACE) inhibitory activity of hetero-chitooligosaccharides prepared from partially different deacetylated chitosans. *Journal of Agricultural and Food Chemistry*, 51, 4930–4934.

Park, P.-J., Je, J.-Y., and Kim, S.-K. (2003b). Free radical scavenging activity of chitooligosaccharides by electron spin resonance spectrometry. *Journal of Agricultural and Food Chemistry*, 51, 4624–4627.

Park, P.-J., Je, J.-Y., and Kim, S.-K. (2004). Free radical scavenging activities of differently deacetylated chitosans using an ESR spectrometer. *Carbohydrate Polymers*, 55, 17–22.

Park, P.-J., Lee, H.-K., and Kim, S.-K. (2004). Preparation of hetero-chitooligosaccharides and their antimicrobial activity on *Vibrio parahaemolyticus*. *Journal of Microbiology and Biotechnology*, 14, 41–47.

Park, S.-G., Lee, D.-Y., Seo, S.-K., Lee, S.-W., Kim, S.-K., Jung, W.-K., Kang, M.-S., Choi, Y. H., Yea, S. S., and Choi, I. (2008). Evaluation of anti-allergic properties of caffeic acid phenethyl ester in a murine model of systemic anaphylaxis. *Toxicology and Applied Pharmacology*, 226, 22–29.

Park, Y. J., Lee, W. C., Yim, H. W., and Park, Y. M. (2007). The association between sleep and obesity in Korean adults. *Journal of Preventive Medicine and Public Health, Yebang Uihakhoe chi*, 40, 454–460.

Park, Y. L., Kim, H. D., Kim, K. H., Kim, M. N., Kim, J. W., Ro, Y. S., Park, C. W., Lee, K. H., Lee, A. Y., and Cho, S. H. (2006). Report from ADRG: A study on the diagnostic criteria of Korean atopic dermatitis. *Korean Journal of Dermatology*, 44, 659–663.

Porst, H., Rosen, R., Padma-Nathan, H., Goldstein, I., Giuliano, F., and Ulbrich, E. (2001). The efficacy and tolerability of vardenafil, a new, oral, selective phosphodiesterase type 5 inhibitor, in patients with erectile dysfunction: The first at-home clinical trial. *International Journal of Impotence Research*, 13, 192.

Prudden, J. F., Migel, P., Hanson, P., Friedrich, L., and Balassa, L. (1970). The discovery of a potent pure chemical wound-healing accelerator. *The American Journal of Surgery*, 119, 560–564.

Qian, Z.-J., Jung, W.-K., Byun, H.-G., and Kim, S.-K. (2008). Protective effect of an antioxidative peptide purified from gastrointestinal digests of oyster, *Crassostrea gigas* against free radical induced DNA damage. *Bioresource Technology*, 99, 3365–3371.

Qian, Z.-J., Jung, W.-K., and Kim, S.-K. (2008). Free radical scavenging activity of a novel antioxidative peptide purified from hydrolysate of bullfrog skin, *Rana catesbeiana Shaw*. *Bioresource Technology*, 99, 1690–1698.

Rajapakse, N., Jung, W.-K., Mendis, E., Moon, S.-H., and Kim, S.-K. (2005). A novel anticoagulant purified from fish protein hydrolysate inhibits factor XIIa and platelet aggregation. *Life Sciences*, 76, 2607–2619.

Rajapakse, N., Kim, M. M., Mendis, E., and Kim, S. K. (2008). Inhibition of inducible nitric oxide synthase and cyclooxygenase-2 in lipopolysaccharide-stimulated RAW264. 7 cells by carboxybutyrylated glucosamine takes place via down-regulation of mitogen-activated protein kinase-mediated nuclear factor-κB signaling. *Immunology*, 123, 348–357.

Rajapakse, N., Mendis, E., Kim, M.-M., and Kim, S.-K. (2007). Sulfated glucosamine inhibits MMP-2 and MMP-9 expressions in human fibrosarcoma cells. *Bioorganic and Medicinal Chemistry*, 15, 4891–4896.

Ryu, B., Himaya, S., Qian, Z.-J., Lee, S.-H., and Kim, S.-K. (2011). Prevention of hydrogen peroxide-induced oxidative stress in HDF cells by peptides derived from seaweed pipefish, *Syngnathus schlegeli*. *Peptides*, 32, 639–647.

Ryu, B., Kim, M., Himaya, S., Kang, K.-H., and Kim, S.-K. (2014). Statistical optimization of high temperature/pressure and ultra-wave assisted lysis of *Urechis unicinctus* for the isolation of active peptide which enhance the erectile function in vitro. *Process Biochemistry*, 49, 148–153.

Ryu, B. and Kim, S. K. (2013). Potential beneficial effects of marine peptide on human neuron health. *Current Protein and Peptide Science*, 14, 173–176.

Ryu, B., Li, Y., Qian, Z.-J., Kim, M.-M., and Kim, S.-K. (2009). Differentiation of human osteosarcoma cells by isolated phlorotannins is subtly linked to COX-2, iNOS, MMPs, and MAPK signaling: Implication for chronic articular disease. *Chemico-Biological Interactions*, 179, 192–201.

Ryu, B., Qian, Z.-J., Kim, M.-M., Nam, K. W., and Kim, S.-K. (2009). Anti-photoaging activity and inhibition of matrix metalloproteinase (MMP) by marine red alga, *Corallina pilulifera* methanol extract. *Radiation Physics and Chemistry*, 78, 98–105.

Saito, T., Shimazaki, Y., Kiyohara, Y., Kato, I., Kubo, M., Iida, M., and Koga, T. (2004). The severity of periodontal disease is associated with the development of glucose intolerance in non-diabetics: The Hisayama study. *Journal of Dental Research*, 83, 485–490.

Sakamoto, H. (2010). Oral infection disease update. *Dental Care*, 24(4), 5–10.

Schuller-Levis, G., Quinn, M. R., Wright, C., and Park, E. (1994). Taurine protects against oxidant-induced lung injury: Possible mechanism (s) of action. In Huxtable, R. J. and Michalk, D. (Eds.), *Taurine in Health and Disease*, pp. 31–39, Springer, New York.

Schuller-Levis, G. B., Gordon, R. E., Park, E., Pendino, K. J., and Laskin, D. L. (1995). Taurine protects rat bronchioles from acute ozone-induced lung inflammation and hyperplasia. *Experimental Lung Research*, 21, 877–888.

Senthilkumar, K. and Kim, S.-K. (2013). Marine invertebrate natural products for anti-inflammatory and chronic diseases. *Evidence-Based Complementary and Alternative Medicine*, 2013, 1–10.

Senthilkumar, K., Manivasagan, P., Venkatesan, J., and Kim, S.-K. (2013). Brown seaweed fucoidan: Biological activity and apoptosis, growth signaling mechanism in cancer. *International Journal of Biological Macromolecules*, 60, 366–374.

Senthilkumar, K., Venkatesan, J., and Kim, S.-K. (2014). Marine derived natural products for osteoporosis. *Biomedicine and Preventive Nutrition*, 4, 1–7.

Shahidi, F., Kamil, J., Jeon, Y.-J., and Kim, S.-K. (2002). Antioxidant role of chitosan in a cooked cod (*Gadus morhua*) model system. *Journal of Food Lipids*, 9, 57–64.

Shim, S.-Y., Quang-To, L., Lee, S.-H., and Kim, S.-K. (2009). *Ecklonia cava* extract suppresses the high-affinity IgE receptor, FcεRI expression. *Food and Chemical Toxicology*, 47, 555–560.

Siriwardhana, N., Kalupahana, N. S., and Moustaid-Moussa, N. (2012). Health benefits of n-3 polyunsaturated fatty acids: Eicosapentaenoic acid and doco-sahexaenoic acid. In Kim, S.-K. (Ed.), *Advances in Food and Nutrition Research - 65*, pp. 211–222, Academic Press, Cambridge, MA.

Song, N.-Y. and Surh, Y.-J. (2013). Health beneficial effects of docosahexaenoic acid. In Kim, S.-K. (Ed.), *Marine Biomaterials*, pp. 413–436, CRC Press, Boca Raton, FL.

Soskolne, W. A. and Klinger, A. (2001). The relationship between periodontal diseases and diabetes. An overview. *Annals of Periodontology*, 6, 91–98.

South Korean Government. (2012). National population and housing census. http://kostat.go.kr/portal/korea/index.action.

Strachan, D. P. (1989). Hay fever, hygiene and household size. *BMJ*, 299, 1259–1260.

Sugano, M., Fujikawa, T., Hiratsuji, Y., and Hasegawa, Y. (1978). Hypocho-lesterolemic effects of chitosan in cholesterol-fed rats. *Nutrition Reports International*, 18, 531–538.

Sugano, M., Fujikawa, T., Hiratsuji, Y., Nakashima, K., Fukuda, N., and Hasegawa, Y. (1980). A novel use of chitosan as a hypocholesterolemic agent in rats. *American Journal of Clinical Nutrition*, 33(4), 787–793.

Sumiyoshi, M. and Kimura, Y. (2006). Low molecular weight chitosan inhibits obesity induced by feeding a high-fat diet long-term in mice. *Journal of Pharmacy and Pharmacology*, 58, 201–207.

Tachiyashiki, K. and Imaizumi, K. (1993). Effects of vegetable oils and C18-unsaturated fatty acids on plasma ethanol levels and gastric emptying in etha-nol-administered rats. *Journal of Nutritional Science and Vitaminology*, 39, 163–176.

Takahashi, K. and Kaminogawa. (2008). Intestinal microbiota and allergy. *Bioindustry*, 25, 40–47.

Takahashi, Y., Tashiro, Y., and Konishi, K. (2015). Oral Streptococci and systemic diseases. *Bioindustry*, 32, 5–11.

Takeda, T., Majima, M., and Okuda, H. (1998). Effects of chondroitin sulfate from salmon nasal cartilage on intestinal absorption of glucose. *Journal of Japanese Society of Nutrition and Food Science (Japan)*, 51, 213–217.

Tanaka, H., Takekura, H., Watanabe, M. et al. (1985). Effect of taurine on lipolytic activity of adipose tissue in exercise trained rats. *Sulfur Amino Acids*, 8, 481–488.

Theodosakis, J., Buff, S., Adderly, B., and Fox, B. (2004). *The Arthritis Cure: The Medical Miracle That Can Halt, Reverse, and May Even Cure Osteoarthritis*. Macmillan, Basingstroke, UK.

Thomas, N. V. and Kim, S.-K. (2011). Potential pharmacological applications of polyphenolic derivatives from marine brown algae. *Environmental Toxicology and Pharmacology*, 32, 325–335.

Thomas, N. V. and Kim, S.-K. (2013). Beneficial effects of marine algal compounds in cosmeceuticals. *Marine Drugs*, 11, 146–164.

Thomas, N. V., Manivasagan, P., and Kim, S.-K. (2014). Potential matrix metal-loproteinase inhibitors from edible marine algae: A review. *Environmental Toxicology and Pharmacology*, 37, 1090–1100.

Thomas, N. V., Venkatesan, J., Manivasagan, P., and Kim, S.-K. (2015). Production and biological activities of chitooligosaccharides (COS)—An overview. *Journal of Chitin and Chitosan Science*, 3, 1–10.

Tsujita, T., Tsukada, H., Nakao, M., Oshiumi, H., Matsumoto, M., and Seya, T. (2004). Sensing bacterial flagellin by membrane and soluble orthologs of Toll-like receptor 5 in rainbow trout (*Onchorhynchus mikiss*). *Journal of Biological Chemistry*, 279(47), 48588–48597.

United Nations Department of Economic and Social Affairs. (2015). World population project to reach 9.7 billion by 2050. http://www.un.org/en/development/desa/news/population/2015-report.html.

Van Ta, Q., Kim, M.-M., and Kim, S.-K. (2006). Inhibitory effect of chitooligosaccha-rides on matrix metalloproteinase-9 in human fibrosarcoma cells (HT1080). *Marine Biotechnology*, 8, 593–599.

Van Ta, Q., Yoon, M., Yang, H., Kim, J., Cho, S., Kang, K.-H., Kim, Y.-S., Park, S.-J., and Kim, S.-K. (2015). Effects of blue mussel (ME) water extracts on pentobarbital-induced sleep and the sleep architecture in mice. *Food Science and Biotechnology*, 24, 295–300.

Venkatesan, J., Bhatnagar, I., Manivasagan, P., Kang, K.-H., and Kim, S.-K. (2015). Alginate composites for bone tissue engineering: A review. *International Journal of Biological Macromolecules*, 72, 269–281.

Venkatesan, J. and Kim, S.-K. (2010). Chitosan composites for bone tissue engineering—An overview. *Marine Drugs*, 8, 2252–2266.

Vo, T.-S., Kim, J.-A., Ngo, D.-H., Kong, C.-S., and Kim, S.-K. (2012). Protective effect of chitosan oligosaccharides against FcɛRI-mediated RBL-2H3 mast cell activation. *Process Biochemistry*, 47, 327–330.

Vo, T.-S., Kim, J.-A., Wijesekara, I., Kong, C.-S., and Kim, S.-K. (2011). Potent effect of brown algae (*Ishige okamurae*) on suppression of allergic inflammation in human basophilic KU812F cells. *Food Science and Biotechnology*, 20, 1227–1234.

Vo, T.-S. and Kim, S.-K. (2010). Potential anti-HIV agents from marine resources: An overview. *Marine Drugs*, 8, 2871–2892.

Vo, T.-S. and Kim, S.-K. (2013). Fucoidans as a natural bioactive ingredient for functional foods. *Journal of Functional Foods*, 5, 16–27.

Vo, T.-S., Kong, C.-S., and Kim, S.-K. (2011). Inhibitory effects of chitooligosaccha-rides on degranulation and cytokine generation in rat basophilic leukemia RBL-2H3 cells. *Carbohydrate Polymers*, 84, 649–655.

Vo, T.-S., Ngo, D.-H., Kim, J.-A., Ryu, B., and Kim, S.-K. (2011). An antihyper-tensive peptide from tilapia gelatin diminishes free radical formation in murine microglial cells. *Journal of Agricultural and Food Chemistry*, 59, 12193–12197.

Vo, T.-S., Ngo, D.-H., and Kim, S.-K. (2012). Marine algae as a potential phar-maceutical source for anti-allergic therapeutics. *Process Biochemistry*, 47, 386–394.

Vo, T.-S., Ngo, D.-H., Van Ta, Q., and Kim, S.-K. (2011). Marine organisms as a therapeutic source against herpes simplex virus infection. *European Journal of Pharmaceutical Sciences*, 44, 11–20.

Vo, T.-S., Ngo, D.-H., Van Ta, Q., Wijesekara, I., Kong, C.-S., and Kim, S.-K. (2012). Protective effect of chitin oligosaccharides against lipopolysaccharide-induced inflammatory response in BV-2 microglia. *Cellular Immunology*, 277, 14–21.

Watanabe, M., Ono, M., and Minato, K. (1987). Effects of taurine on the metabolism under physical exercise. *Sulfur Amino Acids*, 10, 183–186.

Whitescarver, S. A., Ott, C. E., Jackson, B. A., Guthrie Jr, G. P., and Kotchen, T. A. (1984). Salt-sensitive hypertension: Contribution of chloride. *Science*, 223, 1430–1433.

Whittemore, C. T. and Kyriazakis, I. (2008). *Whittemore's Science and Practice of Pig Production*. John Wiley & Sons, New York.

Wijesekara, I., Pangestuti, R., and Kim, S.-K. (2011). Biological activities and potential health benefits of sulfated polysaccharides derived from marine algae. *Carbohydrate Polymers*, 84, 14–21.

Wijesekara, I., Yoon, N. Y., and Kim, S. K. (2010). Phlorotannins from *Ecklonia cava* (Phaeophyceae): Biological activities and potential health benefits. *BioFactors*, 36, 408–414.

Yamagishi, S.-I. (2017). *Diabetes and Aging-related Complications*. Springer, Beijing, China.

Yamashita, A. and Nishimura, F. (2015). Periodontitis and diabetes mellitus. *Bioindustry*, 28, 53–58.

Yamashita, Y. and Sakamoto, K. (2015). Development of functional peptide in cosmetic industry. *Bioindustry*, 32, 56–63.

Yoon, N. Y., Eom, T.-K., Kim, M.-M., and Kim, S.-K. (2009). Inhibitory effect of phlorotannins isolated from *Ecklonia cava* on mushroom tyrosinase activity and melanin formation in mouse B16F10 melanoma cells. *Journal of Agricultural and Food Chemistry*, 57, 4124–4129.

Yoon, N. Y., Lee, S.-H., and Kim, S.-K. (2009). Phlorotannins from *Ishige okamurae* and their acetyl-and butyrylcholinesterase inhibitory effects. *Journal of Functional Foods*, 1, 331–335.

Zhang, C. and Kim, S.-K. (2009). Matrix metalloproteinase inhibitors (MMPIs) from marine natural products: The current situation and future prospects. *Marine Drugs*, 7, 71–84.

Zhang, C., Li, X., and Kim, S.-K. (2012). Application of marine biomaterials for nutraceuticals and functional foods. *Food Science and Biotechnology*, 21, 625–631.

Zhang, C., Li, Y., Qian, Z.-J., Lee, S.-H., Li, Y.-X., and Kim, S.-K. (2011). Dieckol from *Ecklonia cava* regulates invasion of human fibrosarcoma cells and modulates MMP-2 and MMP-9 expression via NF-κB pathway. *Evidence-Based Complementary and Alternative Medicine*, 2011, 1–8.

Zhang, C., Li, Y., Shi, X., and Kim, S.-K. (2010). Inhibition of the expression on MMP-2, 9 and morphological changes via human fibrosarcoma cell line by 6, 6'-bieckol from marine alga *Ecklonia cava*. *BMB Reports*, 43, 62–68.

Zhang, E., Kim, J.-J., Shin, N., Yin, Y., Nan, Y., Xu, Y., Hong, J., Hsu, T. M., Chung, W., and Ko, Y. (2017). High omega-3 polyunsaturated fatty acids in fat-1 mice reduce inflammatory pain. *Journal of Medicinal Food*, 20, 535–541.

Zou, Y., Li, Y., Kim, M.-M., Lee, S.-H., and Kim, S.-K. (2009). Ishigoside, a new glyceroglycolipid isolated from the brown alga *Ishige okamurae*. *Biotechnology and Bioprocess Engineering*, 14, 20–26.

Zou, Y., Qian, Z.-J., Li, Y., Kim, M.-M., Lee, S.-H., and Kim, S.-K. (2008). Antioxidant effects of phlorotannins isolated from *Ishige okamurae* in free radical mediated oxidative systems. *Journal of Agricultural and Food Chemistry*, 56, 7001–7009.

# Index

Note: Page numbers followed by f and t refer to figures and tables respectively.

Printed and bound by CPI Group (UK) Ltd, Croydon, CR0 4YY

17/10/2024

01775660-0007